Health and Fitness confidential

The Best kept secret of fitness industry

Copyright 2015 © Kate Philips

Introduction

Fitness is the ultimate goal of every one who want to live a healthy lifestyle. This book will tackle the most crucial questions that everyone want to know, what makes one fit? What makes one to achieve long lasting fitness? What are the factors to determine if the person fit or not? This essential questions are the questions that will be tackled in this book and answered in the most convenient way as possible.

Obesity has become a global problem now-a-days. It has spread like an epidemic all over the world. More than 1.5 billion people are suffering from obesity worldwide. Moreover, one third and above of adults in the US are obese. The main reason for such a widespread condition is unhealthy lifestyle and food. Having a fit body is considered an unachievable dream by many among us. Why it is so important to us to have a fit body?

Having a fit body not only gives us confidence in every aspect of our lives, but also provides the groundwork for a lifestyle, which keeps most of lifestyle related ailments at a distance from us. Some people believe that having a fit body or fat body only depends on luck and is granted to us. Although this theory has some scientific base in the form of fast and slow metabolism individuals, but it is not entirely true. Fitness and good physique is not a state that is achieved, but rather it is a lifestyle that we have to live continuously.

This might seem daunting that we have to work to be fit every day, but if you really think about it, it's the life you will be living and believe me that it will not be that hard once you are motivated to achieve a healthy and fit physique. It will be just like living a normal life, but making it better and healthier, and will only be a matter of time that you will not even feel like you are working for it. With time, it will be like a normal routine for you.

Keeps most of lifestyle related ailments at a distance from us. Some people believe that having a fit body or fat body only depends on luck and is granted to us. Although this theory has some scientific base in the form of fast and slow metabolism individuals, but it is not entirely true. Fitness and good physique is not a state that is achieved, but rather it is a lifestyle that we have to live continuously. This might seem daunting that we have to work to be fit every day, but if you really think about it, it's the life you will be living and believe me that it will not be that hard once you are motivated to achieve a healthy and fit physique. It will be just like living a normal life, but making it better and healthier, and will only be a matter of time that you will not even feel like you are working for it. With time, it will be like a normal routine for you

Maintaining a healthy weight is important for overall health. It helps prevent many prevalent disease like hypertension, diabetes, cardiovascular problems, gallstones and even certain cancers. Moreover, having a healthy weight gives you confidence and makes you feel good about yourself. Life with good physique will be comparatively more joyful for every human being on this planet.

It is absolutely possible to lose weight and reach an ideal mass; don't find an excuse that it is not impossible so that you may not have to work for it. It won't happen in the blink of an eye, but it will happen eventually. Reaching and maintaining an ideal weight is a harmony between food and activity. You will need some balance between intake and utilization of food and some attitude, motivation and self-control. The key is not some changes in your diet for a short span of time, but you have to make changes in your lifestyle, including healthy eating, regular physical activity and a balance between intake and consumption of calories.

Chapter 1: What makes a person Fit?

Body Mass Index

This is the basic factor you need to know in determining if you're fit or not. What is obesity and overweight? Overweight is having extra body weight from muscle, fat or bone. Obesity is having a high amount of extra body fat. Body mass index is a useful measure of obesity and fitness. Although 'weight' alone can also be used as a unit for those who are trying to maintain a better physical health, but BMI (Body Mass Index) is a better alternative to measuring only weight as it also includes the measures of ones height.

Basic Metabolic Rate (BMR)

Males = 66 + (6.23 x body weight in pounds) + (12.7 x height in inches) – (6.8 x age in years)

Female = 655 + (4.3 x weight in pounds) + (4.7 x height in inches) – (4.7 x age in years)

This will give you your basic metabolic rate or the number of calories you need just to stay alive.

Active Metabolic Rate (AMR)

To work out your active metabolic rate you now need to take the basic metabolic rate and multiply it by one of the number below depending on which one applies to you.

1.1 – Sedentary Physical Activity

1.2 – Light Physical Activity

1.3 – Moderate Physical Activity

1.4 – High Physical Activity

Once you have your Active Metabolic Rate (AMR) number you can begin to work out how many calories you can burn in a day. You now need to add the number of calories burnt through running to the AMR and that's your daily burn. Simply subtract the amount of calories eaten through food and you have your calorie burn for the day.

Body Types

Knowing your body types is essential in determining what kind of diet you need to take. There are basically three body types the Endomorph, the Mesomorph and the Ectomorph.

The Endomorph. This is basically characterized by predominance of body fat. Making the body more bulky in structure. This are the typical people who are easily get fat.

The Mesomorph. These body type are also known to be athletic type of body. They have firm body structure, predominantly large bone structure and more muscular in forms. This the ideal body type for everyone who want to look good and fit.

The Ectomorph. This body type is also known as skinny body type. The have lean muscles and thin body structures. They easily lose weight but takes time to gain one.

Understanding Your Metabolism

Your body is like a car and the calories are the necessary fuels that makes your run as it should be. This whole process is what you called metabolism. The higher the amount of calories burned, the less fat you store regardless of whether you exercise or not. However, just how to burn that fat through enhanced metabolism is where the myths come in to play.

The truth is that metabolism isn't just how fast the body burns calories, but also involves two other important components.

1. Catabolism: This refers to the breaking down of chemical bonds in order to release energy in form of calories
2. The other component is anabolism: This refers to the storage of energy in the form of chemical bonds for later use. Energy is stored in form of fats and glucose.

Both processes are equally as important and both control weight loss and your health.

There are things you need to understand in metabolism. These are the facts that will enlighten you to know better how your body works.

Breakfast is not important part of your Meal

In modern times where people often in hurry skipping breakfast is a common occurrence. The majority of diet blogs, magazines, websites, or TV programs suggest that if you skip breakfast, you are unlikely to achieve your weight loss goals. There are claims that eating a large/heavy breakfast helps you eat less and thus prevent occasional binge eating.

Other dieters believe that if you skip breakfast, you'll slow down metabolism and inhibit the burning of calories. That's why you will hear such quotes like eat breakfast like a king, lunch like a prince and dinner as a pauper. Unfortunately, this is all just a myth.

Studies show that there is a link between consuming fewer calories and eating breakfast, but there isn't any link between skipping breakfast with poor metabolism. What studies found is that eating breakfast helps a person be more physically active but doesn't necessarily rev metabolism.

On the contrary, it's possible to still lose weight while you skip breakfast based on a couple of research studies. People who follow intermittent fasting have revealed it's possible to lose weight when fasting. The bottom line is that though skipping breakfast may cause you to binge eat, never force yourself to eat if you aren't hungry. Pay more focus on the quality and quantity of food you eat; ensure that you eat quality food in a timeframe that matches your work plan or schedule.

Eating in Small Amount in Frequent Manner is Good Idea

If you are a health conscious and often search for the internet for an easy answer to lose weight you might encounter the idea that in losing weight effectively you should eat in small amount but in frequent manner. Some diet 'experts' suggest that dieters should consume frequent and healthier meals in order to rev up metabolism and sustain continued weight loss. It's argued that if you constantly supply calories to your system, the metabolism is kept running, thus you can effortlessly loss weight. Even though the theory may work for some dieters, it's not scientifically proven.

In fact, dieters who witness positive results after adopting frequent smaller meals could be under reporting their meal frequency.

A number of research findings have failed to establish a link between metabolic increase and frequent meals. That said; meal frequency cannot accelerate weight loss and if you adopt this strategy, don't hope for overnight results. There are concerns that eating frequent meals could make you eat excess calories and thus gain weight in the process. Focus on overall calorie control and eat plenty of fiber, protein and other micronutrients. The quality of food you eat is more important than frequency of the meals.

Glycaemic Index Matters

Maye you already heard about Glycemic Index but do you know what Glycemic Index really means? Foods, which are usually digested slowly in the body such as nuts, veggies, whole grains, are considered to be of low glycemic index. These foods are recommended to dieters, as they're believed to promote satiety, and fight occasional hunger or cravings.

Foods such as white bread or white rice are said to be in the high glycemic index and thus hamper weight loss process. These foods are blamed for causing insulin or sugar spikes, which trigger cravings and decreased satiety. The argument is that when you consume foods whose nutrients are absorbed quickly into the bloodstream, this leads to increased production of insulin in order to facilitate that movement of such nutrients from the blood into the cells for storage or for energy.

Based on varied scientific studies, there are contradicting results on glycemic index on rate of metabolism and weight loss. One study found out that those men who eat high-glycemic index foods for a month had a lower insulin resistance compared to those on low-glycemic index foods.

Based on the study, the men didn't gain weight with high glycemic index diet contrary to popular belief. On the other hand, a review on 31 different studies didn't come to conclusive findings that low-glycemic foods can suppress appetite. Of these, majority of 16 studies showed contrary results.

Caffeine

Caffeine are known to be weight busters. Research shows that people who take caffeine can burn higher amount of calories compared to those who don't take coffee. Although caffeine can boost metabolism when ingested before exercise, there isn't a metabolic boost that breaks down the empty calories in caffeinated drinks. Based on a study from Mayo Clinic, an energy drink can offer calories that amount to ¼ cup of sugar-which after reaching the body triggers storage of fat.

Researchers found that taking 500mg of green tea extract could boost metabolism by around 2 percent after 4 hours of taking. Based on these finding, green tea extract on its own has minor effect on your metabolism.

If you need to burn calories from drinks, go for 2 tall glasses of tap water. Research shows that 17 ounces of water can boost your metabolism by over 30 percent. A different research found out that if you boost your water intake by 1.5 liters in a day, you'd burn an extra 17,400 calories in a year.

The Truth about Skinner People

Many people always envy skinner people. Skinner people may appear to overeat without a direct impact on their weight, which may make them appear to have a higher metabolism. To your surprise, individuals with bigger bodies have higher metabolism at rest compared to thinner people. If thin, you tend to have slower resting metabolism and thus you'd burn less calories at rest. However, be aware that the amount of muscle directly affects the amount of calories burned. This explains why muscular people tend to have a faster metabolism.

However, skeletal muscle has a low metabolic rate of around 6 calories per pound. Resistance training helps rev metabolism and burn fat but your brainpower has a bigger contribution.

A pound of brain can burn around 109 calories in a day. Research has shown that exercising helps increase size of brain, thus boosts metabolic rate. Although your body size may matter, the body composition has a greater impact on metabolism.

Midnight Snack

Many of us are afraid to eat at night because we believe that it will eventually turn into fat. At rest, the rate of metabolism is said to be low. That's why eating food beyond 8pm is thought to overload the metabolic process. However, it is important to point out that a number of factors like hormones, food content, food quality and your energy expenditure all have a role to play in the storage of fat.

Avoiding eating late at night cannot help prevent storage of fat; your focus should be on what you eat and its quantity. Actually, if you eat high-quality foods in the right serving, you might not notice the difference in eating earlier or late night.

During a research by European Journal of Nutrition, men were put into two groups; one group fed on carbs throughout and the other reserved carbs for late night snack. The people who ate carbs at night were observed to exhibit a higher diet-induced thermogenesis. Thus, they were able to burn more calories throughout the following day. The group that ate carbs throughout the day showed higher levels of blood sugar, and were more likely to become obese. Nighttime carb eaters burned 27 percent more body fat and were 14 percent more satiated than other dieters.

Metabolism and Weight Loss

Metabolism and weight loss have a strong correlation to each other. If you are trying to lose weight, you are likely to be carried away by this myth. The truth is that different scientific studies have shown that, the fatter you are, the higher the rate of resting metabolism, which refers to the calories burned at rest. This means that if you have a bigger body, you will need a higher rate of metabolism to keep the body supplied with calories or energy required. When you are sedentary, you will often burn lesser calories, but this has nothing to do with your lower rate of metabolism.

Controlling your Metabolism

Controlling your metabolism takes enough courage and proper knowledge. If you are overweight, it is common to blame all your weight loss problems on your unpredictable/uncontrollable metabolism. Research shows that you actually have control of your metabolism.

Your ability to burn calories depends on your body composition. This simply means that you can easily burn fat through lifting weights. Various exercise habits and dietary changes can affect how fast you burn calories at rest. Let's take a quick look at some of the things you can do to take charge of your metabolism:

Sleep

Sleep is an essential body cycle. Research has shown that the amount of rest you get at night affects your mood, productivity as well as the rate of metabolism. If you are deprived of sleep, you tend to have lower control on blood glucose levels.

Rehydrated

Our body is mainly composed of water. Drinking enough water in a day can help boost the calories burned, as water triggers thermogenesis. The body is made to burn more calories in a bid to warm up the water to body temperature. If you remain hydrated, you reduce calorie intake (water is filling) and can facilitate higher metabolism during exercise.

Proteins

More proteins means lean body. Taking a high protein diet can help you to expend more energy during its breakdown given that proteins require more energy to break down. This ultimately enhances metabolism.

Now that we've busted the myths you might be having about boosting metabolism, you might now be asking yourself; what truly drives your metabolism? What should you do to supercharge your metabolism to lose weight?

There is no great magic to boosting or revving up the metabolism. What we want to do is to optimize our body's metabolism (and all of its functions) by providing it with a healthy lifestyle. This includes indulging in the best and healthiest foods and the many factors such as enough sleep, pure water, clean air and sunshine that will help give the body the best chance of achieving optimal health.

Chapter 2: The Problem of Obesity

What makes people susceptible to Obesity?

There are many factors that can cause obesity. Obesity is defined as the abnormal gain of weight due to the accumulation of the fats in the body. A person is called obese when he gains weight that is greater than the standard range with respect to his height. Of course, this is not a healthy condition for anyone, and is among the major concerns now-a-days worldwide as it may lead to many other diseases and health problems. The standard range that shows a standard measure of weight-for-height is called as BMI (Body Mass Index). As described before, if BMI of a person is calculated to be 30 or above, the person is called obese. The normal range for BMI is 25 and people falling within this range, are said to have normal weight to height ratio. So, you can easily determine whether you are having a normal physique or slowly inclining towards obesity. World Health Organization concluded that obesity has nearly doubled in the past 30 years and is triggered by a number of factors. The 2008 statistics clearly shows that more than 500 million people are obese, among which, 300 million are women and 200 million men.

Here are the main factors which are concerned as the potential triggers of obesity.

1. Inappropriate Diet

What you eat makes most of what you are. The foremost reason behind obesity is none other than an improper diet. Life has become so busy and hectic for everyone these days. The work schedules do not allow to eat healthier as everyone is in rush for the work and finds it easier to grab a pack of fast food in lunch or dinner without thinking of the consequences. Fast food is usually rich of too many calories, which adds more fat to your body, and turns your body into improper mass. Poor diet and poor lifestyle leads to the development of obesity with time. The poor diet may contain the following, which must be avoided and replaced with healthy, full of vitamins and minerals rich food.

Processed food with large amounts of fats and sugar should be avoided and replaced with fresh cooked vegetables. Alcohol intake leads to accumulation of a large amount of fats as alcohol is rich in calories, thus increase the body weight abnormally. Eating desserts after every meal leads to obesity as desserts have a lot of sugar. Eating more than required also makes your body save fats and turns your body out of shape. Eating junk food is one of the basic potential triggers of obesity.

For enjoying a healthy and diseases-free life, it is important to avoid all the above habits, and adapt healthy eating practice. For maintaining a normal health, it is necessary to take 2000 to 2500 calories per day. People who take more than this amount of calories become obese as body saves all the extra calories in the form of fats.

Dormant Lifestyle

Dormant lifestyle or inactivity is one of the major factors of fat accumulation. . Generally, people consume a lot of calories and are unable to burn them properly because of the lack of activity. So, these calories ultimately get stored in the body as fats and this storage of fats leads to obesity with time. People who work in offices rarely do any physical activity. They need to work all day in a sitting posture, which is one of the main causes of storage of the calories they consume. If a person is not doing any regular exercise, nor he prefers walking or cycling over riding the car or motorbike, he is not doing any physical activity and may develop obesity with time.

Heredity

Obesity often runs in family. Of course, genes are responsible to decide for us. Certain genes are triggered with specific age and environmental factors, when they are already present. It means that the chances of development of obesity in the child of obese parents are more as compared to the child who has lean parents. But, this does not depend entirely on genetics. The researches have proved that the genes for obesity are only triggered when the environmental factors are favorable for their expression, and the environmental factors here are no other than the eating habits. Poor eating habits may develop the disease in the child of obese parents, but, may not develop it in the child of lean parents. So, when it's in your genes, you have to be more concerned and careful with your diet and eating habits to avoiding building up extra body mass.

Health Factors

Health factors is one of the contributors in obesity. Researches have brought many medicines and ailments into concern that are responsible in the development of obesity.

Smoking

Withdrawal symptoms from quitting smoking can also cause obesity... In this condition, weight is gained as a side effect for the stoppage of smoking, and person may develop obesity. There are two reasons behind this weight gain. First is the sensation of taste. As it become better for all the foods, person starts eating a large quantity of it. Second reason is the burning of fewer calories after the stoppage of intake of nicotine. This may be justified by the fact that nicotine is responsible to higher the rate of burning calories, and when a person has suddenly stopped intake of nicotine, the calories burning process slows down, which ultimately leads to obesity. However, smoking is injurious to health and should be quitted to maintain the quality of life.

Cushing syndrome

It is a rare disorder that affects the adrenal glands and the production of cortisone which makes the diseased person obese.

Medicines

Not only medical condition can cause obesity. There are certain medicines that are actively involved in causing obesity, which include the medicines for diabetes, epilepsy, antidepressants, corticosteroids, drugs taken for treatment of schizophrenia, etc. All these medicines intake contribute to weight gain, leading to obesity with time.

Hypothyroidism

Hyperthyroidism is a condition that affects thyroid glands. It is the lack of the proper activity of the thyroid gland, which leads to the deficient production of thyroid hormone. In this condition, it is noticed that the body become abnormally large due to the improper regulation of the calories.

Age

Many people are often susceptible to obesity depending on their age group. Age is yet another important factor that leads to obesity. Aging leads to the loss of muscles, especially when there is little activities in life. As a result, muscles loss leads to the decrease in the amount of burnt calories as the whole process is affected and decelerates. So, with the increase of age, if the calories intake is not reduced, the person may gain weight and develop obesity.

Obesity and Women

Obesity is common troublesome among women. One of important reasons of weight gain in women is the menopause with age. Women normally gain 5pounds of weight at this stage and develop a dense fat layer around their waist. Yet another important reason is the pregnancy in women. During pregnancy, usually women gain weight as the child is developing and this is the need for the child. But, after giving birth to the baby, they need to breast feed the baby and are unable to maintain their weight back to the normal weight. So, after a few pregnancies, usually women develop enough fats, and become obese.

Sleep

Sleep is essential in everyday life. Lack of sleep is also one of the potential causes of obesity as this habit makes person eat more high caloric food, which leads to the accumulation of fats in the body. Sleep helps to regulate a few of the important hormones, including ghrelin, leptin, and insulin. If these hormones are not properly regulated, a person may develop diabetes and obesity. So, In a nutshell, weight gain can be evaded by taking precautionary measures, which include mostly the ways to evade these risk factors. To enjoy a proper healthy life, it is very important to monitor your weight to standard levels, hence you can live a happy natural life forever.

Ideal body Weight.

Many people are dreaming to have a body like a super model. Why is being skinny admirable? What are the benefits of having and maintaining a proper body mass? These are the questions that can be answered very easily with logic. Having a control of your weight ensures good health for the individual for present, and also while he ages on. Over the years, many people gain weight without even noticing, and before they realize they are overweight, become obese enough that they cannot find the right amount of time and energy to become slender again. Sticking to a healthy lifestyle and healthy food is important to avoid getting fat over time. Having a slender body is really good for the health. People having a normal body weight are at a reduced risk for many dangerous disease like diabetes, hypertension, cardiovascular problems, stroke, arthritis, gall stones, infertility, asthma, sleep apnea, snoring, cataracts etc. Slender body and normal body weight gives you a confidence about your body and appearance. Although, it is also important to feel confident about yourself irrespective of your body weight and physical appearance, but, it is also equally important to become of normal weight and feel even more positive about yourself.

Obesity and Calories

Many people believe that obesity is often cause by obesity. Weight gain is due to a very simple and interesting fact that the amount of weight gain is equal to the difference of calories intake and calories utilized. Weight change = calories in – calories out If you eat as much calories in a day as you burn, weight gain will be zero. But, if you eat more calories than you burn, they are deposited in your body, hence de-shaping your body and increasing your weight drastically.

Decreasing the quantity of food taken per day and shifting towards less processed foods helps with weight loss. Shifting towards a diet with more vegetables and fruits have a proven record in weight loss. The quantity of food in your diet is a major factor in deciding your obesity. Although change in type of food is important, but eating a lot of quality food is also not recommended. Reducing quantity of food in general, be it healthy or unhealthy, is the key. By reducing the quantity of food in your everyday life, you are forcing your body to utilize the stored calories for routine bodily functions. Some people tend to gain more weight as compared to others, even though they eat almost same quantities as others. This is because of some genetic predisposition to obesity, but it is not so severe that a little effort cannot mitigate it.

The second important decider in weight gain is lack of activity and lack of exercise. The less your body moves, the less calories it utilizes. Sitting makes you fatter than standing, while standing makes you fatter than walking, and so on. The more physical activity means the more consumption of calories up to the point when stored calories from body starts to consume by our body. Avoid watching a lot of television or sitting at a computer as this promotes little to no activity at all. Third factor contributing in weight gain is the lack sleep. Researchers studied people on same diet with different sleeps concluded that people with less sleep tend to gain more weight.

Aim for the Goal

Losing Weight is an easy feat. There is no shortcut to achieving an ideal body weight. There is no magic food to reduce weight overnight. There is no magic exercise either. This doesn't mean it cannot be achieved. Achieving a healthy body weight is a combination of some lifestyle changes like moving towards healthy food, avoiding high carbohydrates food and doing regular physical activity. The more important thing is to keep a positive attitude that it quite possible with little practice.

Powerful Tips to Lose Weight

Here are some of the following tips by which you can counter the negativity in your life and achieve a perfect body shape that will make your personality stand out of the crowd.

Healthy Living

Losing Weight and Healthy living is often correlates to each other. Healthy diet is very important in trying to achieve a lower body weight. Some people believe the low carbohydrate diet works better than low fat diet. Actually it's the balance between two, both carbohydrates and fats needs to be reduced. The quantity of food also plays a key role.

A lot of good food will still lead to gain in weight. So, to maintain a proper balance, the quantity of food needs to be reduced because they also give in calories to our body. Eating fewer calories is the main strategy under healthy diet. For starters, try to decrease at least 500 calories from your daily intake. The amount of a food being processed is also crucial.

The more something is processed, makes it more unnatural and unhealthier to the body. For example, you will gain less weight eating peanuts than will gain while eating peanut butter. Eating whole grain is more beneficial than eating refined grain. Similarly, whole wheat should be preferred than eating refined wheat bread. Slow foods should be preferred to fast foods. Home cooked meals are much better than restaurants and specially fast foods.

Decrease consumption of fast food to maximum two times per month. Carbonated beverages are the most resilient factors in people gaining weight. The corporations have designed their sodas with formulas that are difficult to remove from our diet. A single Can of soda gives calories, which are consumed by 20 minutes of jogging, and it's a lot of calories. You must get rid of carbonated drinks for your diet plan to work.

Water

Experts agree that water consumption increases the rate at which our body burn calories. The procedure requires an adequate supply of water in order to function efficiently and dehydration slows down the fat-burning process. Burning calories creates toxins, which are removed out of our body with the help of water. Water helps maintain muscle tone by assisting muscles to contract, hence are very useful in lubricating your joints. It is also believed that appropriate hydration can help reduce muscle and joint soreness when exercising. Drinking plenty of water is recommended.

Alcoholic Drinks

Alcohol consumption can affect your weight. Alcohol should be used only moderately. Excess alcohol intake have very negative effects on weight loss. Our body uses alcohol as its fuel and burns alcohol instead of other carbohydrates Alcohol should be used only moderately. Excess alcohol intake have very negative effects on weight loss. Our body uses alcohol as its fuel and burns alcohol instead of other carbohydrates and fats. Therefore, the body is ended up storing carbohydrates and fats from diet in body and burning the alcohol.

By countering all these negativity from your life, eventually, you will choose a healthy and happy life for yourself.

Chapter 3: Eat what makes you Healthy.

Eating is an essential activity for survival. It does not only serves as survival activity but also as a social activity. Eating is such an interesting and unique topic because it's so broad—there are so many types of foods that you can eat, there's so many ways prepare them, and there are foods that are good for you and foods that are bad. Our diets are important because they play a major role in our health. If you maintain a healthy diet and exercise, chances are that you will have good health. If you don't really watch what you eat or you don't exercise regularly, your health could probably use some help.

Another thing that many of us have in common is a limited amount of time. For many people, scheduling meals into their days is a real challenge. Many people fall into the habit of eating unhealthy foods because they are quick, easy, and readily available. However, most foods that you can easily pop into the microwave or eat right out of the package are filled with sugar, calories, trans fats, carbohydrates, high sodium levels, preservatives and other things that are bad for your body. They very rarely contain healthy minerals and nutrients. Although these kinds of foods are easy to eat and do not require much preparation, they come with many drawbacks.

Unhealthy foods can make us overweight and out of shape. They are also known to cause many diseases and conditions. Unfortunately, many corporations try to make their food as tasty and addictive as possible, worrying more about profits than the health of their customers. The most common disease that unhealthy foods can bring on is obesity.

Obesity is a relevant and climbing problem in the United States. Studies suggest that at least 42% of our population will be obese by the year 2050—that's almost half of society! Doctors and researchers have linked obesity with other health complications such as heart disease and diabetes. Unhealthy eating can also lead to depression because your diet can affect your hormonal balance. The high sodium content in unhealthy foods can lead to kidney, liver, heart, and blood pressure complications.

All in all, unhealthy eating can lead to nutritional deficiencies that can ultimately cause low energy, sleep problems, mood swings, and a hindered concentration. It is also easier to get injured with an unhealthy diet, it is easier to fall victim to sickness and it takes longer for your body to recover from these things.

It is important to eat healthy because good foods can provide your body with enough vitamins, minerals, and nutrients that it needs to function. By starting off on the right foot, you can avoid becoming obese and can avoid many unpleasant medical problems in the future. Healthy eating can make you feel upbeat, motivated, and energetic, which is important for living a fulfilling life.

Healthy eating also pays off because it can strengthen your body against certain diseases, such as type 2 diabetes, heart disease, certain cancers, and heart disease. Healthy eating is essential for many aspects of our health and it sets a good example for your friends and family, especially the children in your life.

Healthy eating has many obvious benefits. It can help you control your weight and your appearance because you will not be consuming as much food that has a high fat and calorie count. Healthy foods can also fill you just as fast as unhealthy foods, so your chances of overeating may decrease.

It can help you manage your blood sugar level and reduce your chances of developing type 2 diabetes because healthy foods do not contain as much sugar as traditional unhealthy foods. Healthy foods contain many antioxidants and low levels of cholesterol, which can help protect and strengthen your heart so that you can live a long, healthy life.

There are also some little-known benefits of eating healthy, which many people are not aware about. Eating healthy can help strengthen your teeth, fend off bad breath, reduce your chances of developing gum disease, reduce the amount of wrinkles on your skin, make you more productive, and it can keep your stress levels low. It can also prevent bloating, constipation, mood swings, and cravings. It can even make you more knowledgeable because it requires educating yourself to eat healthy. As you can see, there are more benefits to eating healthy than to eating unhealthy. It can positively affect almost every part of your body.

In a nutshell, think of this way: as long as you stay healthy, your chances of living longer and happier improve. You can live long enough to raise and support a family, you will save money by not having too many doctor visits, you can be happier, you can get more done, and people can look up to you as a healthy role model.

Some people confuse the idea of eating healthy as being on a diet. The truth is that eating healthy is not the same thing as being on a diet—people tend to only stay on diets for a certain amount of time—eating healthy is something that you should begin doing as soon as possible and you should continue to do it for the rest of your life.

Make sure your goals have a powerful that will truly motivate you to act consistently. For example, if you want to lose weight and gain strength… why do you want to do that? Is it so you can feel better about yourself? Is it so that you will be able to compete at a higher level? Is it because you want to be more attractive to the opposite sex? Is it so that you can live longer and happier with the people you love?

Make sure your reason is compelling, something that truly motivates you, and remind yourself of it often. Most importantly, have fun! Changing your lifestyle in terms of health means that you get to try out new recipes, activities, and exercises, so have some fun with it and enjoy the process. Be sure to review your weight loss goals daily and use some visualization to see yourself in the healthy state of being that you want to be in.

Chapter 4: What You Should Eat

What you eat matters. It clearly defines whether you will be fit or not. There are known foods that supplement each other needs in terms of caloric contents. Some foods promotes losing weight like these foods listed here.

Turmeric

Turmeric is known for its spicy textures and a well-known spice, commonly used in Asian cooking. It is a rhizome, which means the part of the plant we consume is the rootstock. Turmeric is a member of the ginger family and is deep yellow to orange in color. It has been shown over the years to have significant benefits in terms of health, including being one of the most powerful natural anti-inflammatories there is. It also doesn't produce any of the side effects that many drugs do and can also help-to alleviate the risks of ulcerative colitis.

Turmeric is particularly useful for those with arthritic or rheumatic conditions. It helps to prevent the oxidization of cholesterol, stopping plaque from building up in the arteries and can also stop the growth of cancer cells. In terms of nutrition, turmeric is a valuable source of vitamin B6, fiber, potassium, manganese and iron. It can be taken fresh or in capsule form. It should be mixed with a little black pepper, as this will increase the absorption of the turmeric in the body by around 2000%.

Oysters

A popular seafood delicacy oyster often served in dinner gathering. Other than a delicacy it is also packed with vitamins and minerals.

These nutrients can help with weight loss, increase the rate of tissue growth and repair, boost metabolism, balance out cholesterol levels, cut blood pressure, help with healing of wounds, improve the immune system and promote healthy growth. If that weren't enough, they are also a very powerful aphrodisiac, can help to strengthen bones and improve blood circulation.

Oysters contain a very high number of minerals, organic compounds and vitamins with zinc being one of the most prominent. They also have high protein levels, vitamins B12, D and C, iron, manganese, copper, selenium, thiamin, niacin, riboflavin, potassium, sodium and phosphorus. Finally, oyster are also an excellent source of antioxidants, good cholesterol, water and omega 3 fatty acids.

Soy

Soy is also known as superfood for its wide variety of uses. Fermented soy covers a wide range of foods, including tempeh, miso, natto and tamari. By fermenting soybeans, we have a food that is packed full of nutrients instead of being hazardous to health, which soybeans can be in their unfermented form. As a bean, soy is full of protein and the process of fermentation breaks the proteins down into constituent amino acids, allowing for easier absorption in the digestive system. Glutamic acid and leucine are fond in abundance in all forms of fermented soy. Leucine is used for helping to build up muscles while the glutamic acid is used for neurotransmission, particular in the brain's cognitive areas. Both natto and tempeh contain high levels of proline and serine, both of which are amino acids. Proline supports the production of collagen and serine supports the nervous system.

Also broken down by the fermentation process are oligosaccharides, which are known to cause indigestion and gas. Phytic acid is also reduced – this acid is responsible for reducing proper absorption of nutrients and minerals in some people – the fermentation virtually eliminates it, meaning you get more of the benefits of the minerals in the soy.

Broth

Broth are known to be a good source saturated fats. Drinking broth made from boiled bones is nothing new and it is possibly one of the cheapest forms of nutrition there is. Bone broth is incredibly healthy, tastes amazing and can be used in a number of ways, including soups, sauces, and gravies and to cook vegetables and grains in.

Bones are cooked in water and all the minerals, like phosphorus, magnesium, calcium and many other nutrients and trace minerals leach out into the water, which is easily absorbed in your body. Bone broth also contains chondroitin and glucosamine, which are recommended for mitigating arthritis and pains in the joints. Bones also contain a high level of gelatin, a cheap way of gaining supplementary protein, which provides support for the connective tissues, hair, skin and nails.

Coconut Oil

Popular in the tropics coconut is a staple food for some tropical countries. Coconut oil is made from the kernel or meat of a mature coconut and is quickly gaining popularity as a remedy for many different health issues. For a long time it was seen as an unhealthy fat but constant research is showing it to be one of the best oils for human health. It has been shown to help in the reduction of abdominal fat if it is used as part of a low carbohydrate, high fat diet. The fatty acids found in coconut oil help to curb the appetite, providing a significant reduction in the amount of food eaten. The

MCT (medium chain triglyceride) in coconut oil has also been shown to improve the way energy is expended and to assist the body in becoming efficient at fat burning. They also help the ketones in the body to increase, providing an alternate energy source for the brain. Coconut oil also contains vitamins A and E, physterols and polyphonold, all of which provide a strong antioxidant activity and reduce the risks of strokes and heart diseases.

Coconut milk comes from the meat of a mature coconut and is very creamy in texture, with a sweet taste. It is often used in cooking and drunk on its own. It contains a high level of saturated fats which, because they are water soluble and ae transported easily from the small intestine, convert to ketones which are the used for energy. Because pretty much all of the MCT is utilized, there is very little, if any, left over that can be deposited in your fat cells. Coconut milk has been shown to be beneficial for those with cognitive disorders as well as providing the brain with energy.

Do try to buy coconut milk that is packaged in cartons or in cans that are clearly marked as BPA free. Most cans are lined with BPS – bisphenol A –, which is a synthetic compound that leaches into the milk. BPA has been widely associated with cancers that are dependent on hormones, such as breast or prostate. High BPA levels in the urine can also lead to peripheral arterial disease and cause a resistance to insulin, which could lead to diabetes.

Avocado

Avocado is known for its high fat content and known as dieter enemy. However, the fat content is of the good variety and does amazing things to the human body Monounsaturated fat is the highest content, perhaps as much as 30 grams per avocado, and this has been shown to reduce triglyceride levels. This makes them good for people with diabetes – eating one or two per day can see triglyceride levels fall by as much as 20%.

Avocado is also a god source of folate with around 28% of the daily recommended amount in just one fruit. As well as supporting the health of the nerve endings and brain function, folate is excellent for pregnant women as it helps to prevent abnormalities in the brain and spine of the developing baby. Another nutrient that the avocado contains in high levels is potassium, which is vital to good muscle contraction as we as helping to prevent high blood pressure and osteoporosis.

Eggs

Natural raised hens that are allowed to freely range are the best source of excellent eggs. Free-range eggs come from hens that are allowed to range freely rather than being cooped up in cages all day long. They also tend to eat food that is organic rather than being fed on foods that are full of chemicals and growth hormones.

Eggs contain a complete protein, which means that all 9 essential amino acids are contained in it. As well as these, there are other sources of protein in eggs that are highly beneficial to the human body. Ovalbumin is found in the egg white and there are also varying levels of B vitamins and vitamins A, D and E. Choline, a B-complex vitamin, is present in abundance and this is used by the body to support cell membranes, stopping a buildup of fat on the liver and for transmitting nerve signals. Niacin is another B vitamin that is found in the egg white and vitamins A, D and E, all of which are fat soluble, can be found in the yolk Perhaps more importantly, 100 grams of whole egg contains around 109 mg of omega-3 essential fatty acids.

Ginger

Ginger and turmeric are close related spices Ginger is powerful anti-inflammatory, effectively stopping nitric oxide in the body from turning into peroxynitrate, a highly damaging free radical. It can help to alleviate pain and swelling associated with arthritis, joint and muscle pains and any other pain or soreness associated with the muscles or joints. It has been shown to wipe out ovarian cancer cells and colorectal cancer cells. Ginger can help to alleviate nausea, dizziness and vomiting and is often used by pregnant women as a remedy for morning sickness.

Sweet Potato

Poor man's diet known for its abundance and easy availability, sweet potatoes are a very distant cousin to the white potato and has a starchy sweet taste. Although they are high in carbohydrate content, this is the good version rather than that found in white potatoes and sweet potatoes are often recommended as a replacement for the humble potato in many diets.

Anthocyanin can be found in the sweet potato, a pigment that determines the color of the vegetable. Purple sweet potatoes in particular contain hepatoprotective properties and are good for helping to reduce inflammation and to entice the liver to produce antioxidant enzymes. Purple anthocyanin's also chase free radicals out of the body and have been shown, in studies on rats, to reduce brain inflammation. The studies showed that the purple sweet potato could also be used to reduce oxidative damage in the liver, caused by a diet that is high in cholesterol. The orange sweet potato contains high levels of vitamin A and white skinned sweet potatoes have been shown to help reduce the risks of type 2 diabetes.

Chia Seeds

Chia is an excellent source of omega 3 fatty acids and fiber. Because they are tiny little seeds, they are easy to add to any meal. Studies show that chia seeds help to boost energy, stabilize the blood sugar, lower cholesterol, and help the digestive processes. For such a tiny seed, chia comes with a surprisingly powerful nutritional profile. As well as the omega 3, chi also contains phosphorus, manganese and calcium.

Current research is studying the use of chia to help with type-2 diabetes, mainly because of its ability to slow down digestion and keep blood sugar level. And, because of this, it can also help to fight stubborn belly fat because it fights resistance to insulin. Chia is extremely high in fiber and is an excellent source of protein, particularly to those who are vegan or vegetarian. It also contains tryptophan, which helps to regulate sleep, appetite and improve moods. Chia seeds have also been shown to lower blood pressure and increase the levels of good cholesterol against bad.

Chapter 5: The Wonders of Lemon

Lemon are known to be a wonder fruit and widely used in variety culinary and medical purposes. Lemon with the aid of salt can do incredible things in losing your weight. Here are some of benefits of lemon in your diet.

Immune System Booster

Lemons are known to boost your immune system for it contain a reasonable level of vitamin C and potassium. Drinking lemon water when you get up helps the body absorb those effectively and can also boost your immune system a little. Vitamin C is also good for your adrenal glands and can help to reduce the negative effects of stress.

Aids Healthy Weight

Lemon helps to detoxify your body and flush all the toxins in your body. Drinking enough will increase your metabolism, which leads to faster fat burning and more energy.

By helping flush the body and improve digestion, lemon water can lead to cleaner skin. It also contains Vitamin C, which is needed for collagen production for smooth, healthy skin.

Now let's look at the benefits of drinking Himalayan salt in water first thing in the morning. First of all, to get any benefit from this, you must drink a glass of moderately salty water first, followed by a glass of lightly salted water and it must be first thing in the morning.

Natural Cleanser

Cleanser of liver for it naturally aids your body to metabolize fats and flush toxins in your body. While you sleep, your liver is very active as your body takes the time to restore and regenerate. Drinking lemon water first thing in the morning ensures that your body can do this effectively and there is also research that shows the lemon juice acid stimulates the production of bile and stomach acids.

Adrenal Glands

Flushing excess salts in your body aids the adrenal glands to perform at optimize level. When waking, our body raises our blood pressure so that sufficient blood reaches the brain – this is so you don't black out when you stand up. That increase in pressure also kick starts your body. To do this, the brain calls on the adrenals for help in getting adrenaline out into your system. This is a huge task for those adrenals and they can get stressed out. The salt water raises your blood pressure for a short period of time, thus relieving the pressure on the adrenals. This will result in higher energy levels throughout the day.

A Healthy Digestive System

It helps to cleanse your Digestive tract and expel all the toxins that affects your body. A morning salt flush can also cleanse your GI system and flush out all the stagnant matter. This allows your digestive system to work better, absorbing more of the nutrients from your food while using up loess in the way of energy. Do be aware that this is a cleanse and your system should be well and truly cleaned out in the first week but the benefits are well worth it.

Improves your Digestion

Lemon in warm water helps indigestion problems. It has the effect of flushing out the digestive systems and rehydrating your body. Unless you get up every hour throughout the night, you have probably gone about 8 hours without drinking and have more than likely been sweating through the night. Drinking lemon water first thing in the morning kick starts both your mind and your body.

Hydrating your Body

Lemon can also fully rehydrate your body by helping you to detoxify and cleanse your system from excess salts. You should always do this before you eat, as it can help with digestion, get rid of toxins that make your body sluggish and also improves your skin and mental performance. The water is just a small part of hydration; your body also needs the electrolytes and minerals contained in the Himalayan salt.

Skin Enhancer

Lemon helps to detoxify your body thus this leads to healthier, happier skin. The vitamin C in the lemon also helps with the production of collagen, which helps to keep your skin looking healthy and smooth.

Chapter 6: Effective Ways in Weight Loss

Losing weight is always a hard work and enough determination. However, maintaining the lost weight is a hundred times more difficult! But if you come to think about it, it is very easy. It is a known fact that you gain weight when you cannot burn the calories that you intake. So all you have to do is cut down on your calorie intake. Then why is it such a challenge to lose weight? We undertake diets which include food that is unbearable to eat and some people even resort to starvation. Although these may work, they have an adverse effect on you – physically and mentally – and hence people generally give up. However, there are other methods by which you can lose weight without having to put yourself under too much of stress.

Monitor your Calorie Intake

Monitoring the amount of food you intake especially the calorie amount is essential in losing weight. Everybody refers to this as dieting. It is pretty obvious that if you reduce your calorie intake, you do have the chance of getting rid of those excess calories which will lead to a loss in weight.

Workout

Workout is always an effective way to lose weight and get fit. You sweat while exercising. You will burn more calories. The more calories you burn, the lesser are stored and this will ultimately result in a loss of weight. The most efficient way to attain weight loss is the combination of the above 2. Lesser calories are consumed and more are burned. This will definitely cause a loss in weight if done by the person on a regular basis.

The next chapters discuss seven different exercises that you can use to help you lose weight and also keep yourself fit and healthy. Performing these exercises will ensure that you have a toned body and are rid of all the unhealthy, extra fat. There might be a few exercises that you might not want to do on account of them being difficult. You must remember that it is those exercises that help you keep yourself fit and healthy.

Most people relate exercise to torture. They might not mean it literally, but they do tend to find exercise strenuous. For instance, consider a student who hates mathematics. He will struggle to go through the problems that have been given to him. He will loathe the professor or the teacher. In the same way, a person who is afraid of the term exercise will hate his trainer and also hate the exercises that he must perform. But there are ways to make exercising fun!

Do the exercises at a time that is most suitable to you. Most people are told that they must finish the exercises in the morning. But this is not true. You can perform these exercises any time. The only thing you need to do is not skip them.

Create a schedule to follow. Mix up the exercises to make it more fun. If there is a monotonous schedule, you might get bored and give up.

Only pick the exercises you find most fun! That way you will never skip. If you love bench presses, perform these on a regular basis. You can use different variations that are provided in this book to help keep it more fun!

Listen to music that makes you want to dance. The blood also sings to the tune of the song making you more energetic. You will not tire too soon and will be able to finish the entire set!

Always take a day off. Treat yourself to an exercise free day. Everybody needs a break from doing whatever they love most to avoid getting bored of it. In the same way, you might get bored if you do not give yourself a break.

You might have come across many articles that state that only a particular form of an exercise is the right form for everybody to practice. This is false. It is best for one to have a variation in the way they perform the exercise for the following reasons:

Every human being is different from the other both in mind and body. A variation that might suit one person does not necessarily have to suit the other. The variations that can be used depend on the person's muscles and body structure and also the history of injury.

The next important aspect to consider is why they are performing that variation of the exercise. They might want to increase their strength and fitness for which they might have to use a variation that will help them use their body as a lever. This way they are increasing the force that is placed on the different muscles in the body.

You need to have a variation in your exercises in order to have strength that is well – rounded.

If you stick to a particular variation because it is popular, you are only hurting yourself. It is best to use variations that are perfect for your body stature.

Chapter 7: Planning Your Diet

Planning your diet is essential in losing weight. Many people think of dieting as a quick solution for becoming skinnier or healthier. However, a true diet is not so simple. A better way to define diet is the type and amount of food that you eat within a certain time frame. There are many different kinds of diets that you have probably heard of—the Atkins diet, the Zone diet, the Weight Watchers diet, the South Beach diet, the Raw Food diet, the Mediterranean diet, Paleo Diet, vegetarian diet, vegan diet, and more. These diets all use different strategies and theories to help people lose weight, but the one thing that they all have in common is that they aim to get people into the habit of eating balanced, nutritional meals.

A healthy diet is essentially a healthy lifestyle. The better you eat, the better your body can function. A healthy diet is one that includes food from each food group, since each group by itself cannot provide your body with the proper vitamins, minerals, and nutrients it needs to function. In this chapter, I will explain each food group so you have a better idea of the standard food pyramid. Then I will go over some great tips that you can follow as you start your own diet. You will also read about some very delicious yet healthy recipes you can start off with. Finally, I will talk about the importance of including exercise with your diet.

Food Pyramid

You have probably heard about the food pyramid at one point in your life. Some packages of food have it on their labels but you have more likely learned about it in school. I don't know about you, but it's been a while since I've been a student, and it's easy to forget many of the things that you've learned in health class. I decided to include an overview of the major food groups so that you can refresh your memory and learn about what kind of foods are the best to eat while dieting.

Whole Grains and Nuts

It is important for you to provide your body with at least 3 ounces of whole grains each day. Whole grains are better than refined grains (for example, wheat bread instead of white bread) because whole grains do not lose their bran and wheat germ when they are refined. Most of us are not familiar with this kind of nut. Brazil nuts, although small, pack a hefty nutritional punch, full of proteins, essential nutrients and fats. Although they are very high in calories – 100 gm is approximately 656 calories – that calorific content comes from high levels of monounsaturated fatty acids, which help to raise the levels lf, HDL cholesterol (the good kind). This can help to protect against heart disease and strokes.

Nuts and seeds can be especially helpful in protecting your insides from constipation, a condition that nobody wants to experience, and nuts and seeds are also great for energy. The older you get, the more constipation can be a problem, so it is very important to watch what you eat. Flax seeds in particular are helpful with this condition because of their high fiber content. Almonds, sunflower seeds, and sesame seeds can also serve as a solution to constipation. Try to avoid red meats, dairy, caffeine, processed foods, and sugar, as all these foods can worsen constipation. It is also important to eat a balanced and healthy diet, especially if you have diabetes, which worsen constipation. Prune juice is also an incredible all natural solution and drinking lots of water, smoothies, and fruit and vegetable juices helps tremendously as well. Constipation medicine can get pretty pricey so it can be helpful to turn to alternative solutions.

Brazil nuts also contain vitamin E which is fat-soluble antioxidant needed to keep the cells of the mucosa and skin healthy and protecting them from damage by free radicals. They also contain very high levels of selenium and are the highest natural source. Selenium is a cofactor of glutathane peroxidase, an antioxidant enzyme that can help to fight against some cancers, heart disease and cirrhosis of the liver. As well as all that, Brazil nuts also contain B-complex vitamins, like niacin, thiamin, riboflavin, folates, vitamin B6 and pantothenic acid.

Whole grains are an excellent source of fiber, vitamins, and minerals, which are essential for staying healthy and energetic. Most pastas, cereals, and bread come in whole grain options. You can also look for foods that contain 100% whole grains such as brown rice, corn, wild rice, and oatmeal. The best way to determine if something has whole grains in it is to carefully read the label.

Eating whole grains can help people whose stomachs do not respond well to acidic foods. At least 20% of the people in the United States suffer from a condition like this, which is better known as acid reflux. If you are susceptible to acid reflux and stomach pain, whole grain oatmeal is a great food to add to your diet. It contains plenty of vitamins, it slows down your digestion, and it is not acidic. You can have oatmeal for breakfast, you can incorporate it into breakfast smoothies, or you can have it topped off with fruits and nuts or ground cinnamon to help protect your body from even more ailments and conditions. Besides whole grains, you can also include honey, bananas, apples, ginger, and green tea in your diet. My personal favorite is Aloe Vera juice which has greatly helped with my own stomach problems. Four cups of Aloe Vera Juice a day, preferably 1 cup before each meal, 5 days a week with two days off per week can work wonders. Yoga is also the best type of exercise for those who experience acid reflux.

Fibres

Fibers are essential in proper functioning of human body. Fruits and vegetables are rich in fibers. It is important for you to provide your body with at least five servings of fruit and vegetables each day. They are generally great for you and can protect your body against a myriad of diseases and ailments. Fruits and vegetables are a very good source of nutrients. Studies also show that eating more fruits and vegetables can help protect you against heart disease, certain cancers, and type 2 diabetes. There are many ways to get your daily serving of fruits and vegetables. You can buy them fresh from the market, you can buy them frozen and use them in smoothies, or you can juice them into a delicious drink. Fruits and vegetables also have many great health benefits other than just protecting your body against diseases.

Red chili peppers have been found to be a good vegetable for suppressing your appetite because they contain a compound called Capsaicin. You can add these peppers to your eggs, your steak, your salads, or you can snack on them by themselves. Yellow bell peppers can help you burn fatter and contains three times the amount of vitamin C than oranges. Snacking on strawberries can help whiten your teeth due to their salicylic acid content. Adding beets to your salads can boost your endurance and make your muscles stronger.

Mangoes can help fend off breast cancer because of their polyphenolics, which can inhibit cancer cells. Adding sweet potatoes to your dinner plate can provide you with enough potassium to strengthen your muscles. The zinc in pumpkins and pumpkin seeds can help enhance your memory and hand-eye-coordination. Pineapples can help you reduce bloating because of their enzyme called bromelain, which is very helpful for digestion. The antioxidants found in corn can help protect your eyes and vision. Spinach can improve your complexion, pears can help you keep away hunger pains, and the healthy fats found in avocados can help you combat mood swings.

The natural acids found in plums can help you fend off a cold or virus. The flavonoids found in blueberries can help you focus, concentrate, and think logically. The simple sugars in raisins can give you a burst of natural energy and protect your bones from osteoporosis. The anti-inflammatory compounds found in onions can help protect your teeth against cavities and the high count of vitamin B6 in white potatoes can help lower your chances of developing heart disease.

If vision and eyesight problems run in your family or if you think that you are susceptible to them, some fruits and vegetables can help protect your eyes. Carrots, red onions, sweet potatoes broccoli, Brussels sprouts, spinach, and bell peppers all contain important vitamins and powerful antioxidants that can protect your eyes from cataracts and deterioration while promoting general eye health. Fruits that are good for promoting eye health include kiwi, cantaloupe, peaches, grapefruit, tomatoes, and oranges. Vision and eyesight problems can be hereditary so it is important to incorporate fruits and vegetables into your diet for extra protection. If you work in front of a computer or have a passion for video games, you can also eat plenty of fruits and vegetables to protect yourself from conditions such as glaucoma, myopia, hyperopia, cataracts, eye strain, and aging.

There are many more types of fruits and vegetables that you can add to your diet, but this chapter should give you a good idea of just how important they are to your overall health. Fruits and vegetables are delicious, filling, refreshing, and versatile—you can become very creative when it comes to cooking with these two foods, so you will not have to worry about getting tired of eating them.

You can also get your daily servings of fruits and vegetables by making smoothies. Smoothies are quick and easy to make and you can have them as a meal or as a snack. You are probably familiar with fruit smoothies but did you know that you can even make vegetable smoothies? They are better known as green smoothies. There is an unlimited variety of smoothies you can make, so feel free to mix and match your favorite fruits and vegetables. Here are a few recipes you can try out:

White Meat and Red Meat

Consuming all kinds of meat are very important for your body because these foods all contain protein pork, beef, poultry, fish, and eggs are. Protein helps your body build and repair tissue. These foods also contain important nutrients such as zinc, iron, magnesium, and B vitamins. Health experts recommend that 25% of your diet should include protein-rich foods. When eating meat, be sure to trim it of all its fat and you can optionally take the skin off of the chicken before eating it. I also recommend eating fish at least twice a week because it contains omega-3 fatty acids, which are also beneficial to your health. The best way to eat meat, chicken, and fish is to grill or roast it. Frying it is another option but fried foods are not as good for your health.

Dairy Products

Milk, yogurt, and cheese fall in the category of dairy products. Eating dairy products is a great way to provide your body with calcium and it makes your bones and teeth strong. For the best results, you should try to stick with low-fat dairy products. Vegans can get their sources of calcium through vegetables such as broccoli or cabbage or through vitamin supplements.

Micronutrients

Adding the proper amount of micronutrients like calcium to your diet can protect your body against kidney stones, which is another horrible and very painful condition that nobody wants to experience. Many people end up in the hospital from kidney stones and those who have had them many times describe it as the worst pain that they have ever experienced. If you are prone to dehydration, if you are overweight, addicted to alcohol, adding salt to all of your food, or eating foods that contain high fructose corn syrup, you may be more susceptible to kidney stones. Too much calcium can also cause kidney stones but on the other hand, if you don't provide your body with enough calcium, you may still be at risk. Low fat milk and low fat cheese are two great, calcium-rich foods that you can add to your diet to help fend off kidney stones. Drinking lots of water is also a great way to avoid getting kidney stones. .

Foods to Eat with Caution

Products with high amounts of sugar and fat, such as butter, chocolate, sodas, mayonnaise, cakes, and a variety of other processed foods should only be eaten sparingly. Products that contain high levels of saturated fats, such as cream, margarine, and fried foods should especially be kept to a minimum; although some saturated fats like the ones found in coconut oil can be very good for you

You don't have to completely torture yourself and cut fats and sugars out of your diet forever, but you should try to limit them from your diet. By limiting these types of foods, they will taste even better when you do allow yourself to have them.

Skin Problems

Excess consumption of unnecessary fats and sugar can cause different skin problems like acne. Acne is a breakout on the skin that affects people of all ages. To control acne, it is very important to eat right. Certain foods can trigger the production of hormones and oil (sugar being one of them), while others can promote good skin health (such as vegetables, fruits, and nuts). Acne is not a life-threatening condition but it can make you look unattractive or feel unpleasant. To get rid of it, you can turn to special facial cleaners, acne creams, laser treatment, or a variety of modern medicines, all of which can be costly. Good "food treatments" for clearing up acne include using grapes, cucumbers, honey, lemons and orange peels as all natural facial cleansers because of their antibacterial, acidic, and moisturizing properties.

Chapter 8: What Diet Plans Works for You

Creating a personalized diet plan can help you better address your eating preferences while working around your school or work schedule. It can also serve as a visual or a map, which can make your diet easier to follow.

The first thing you should do when creating a personalized diet plan is reflect upon yourself. The better you know yourself, the better you can figure out what kind of diet plan you need in order to see successful results. There are a couple of basic, key questions that you can ask yourself to start out.

Creating Personalize Diet Plans

First, ask yourself how many meals you would like to eat per day. Some people can get away with eating two meals but others may like to break their meals up. I would highly recommend breaking your meals up into smaller portions and eating 4-5 times per day. Once I started breaking up my meals into smaller, healthier portions is when I noticed a tremendous increase in my overall wellbeing.

When you've figured out how many meals you want to eat per day, you can try to divide the total amount of calories you want to consume each day by the number of meals that you eat each day. For example, if you only want to eat 2,000 calories per day, you can eat 4 meals of 500 calorie or 2 meals of 1,000 calories, or any combination. Here is one tip: you should try to eat at least three meals per day. Eating smaller meals consistently can help prevent overeating and increase overall alertness and energy level. If you are doing strength training and regular exercise, you often times do not even have to count calories, just eat healthy and when you're hungry. Over time this strategy tends to lead towards an athletic and strong body that is not over weight.

Secondly, ask yourself how much time you will be able to spend preparing your meals. If you're not a fan of cooking or if you have a busy schedule, you will have to figure out how you're going to coordinate your meal preparation. This will all depend on your own schedule. For example, it might be better for you to prepare all of your meals in advance on Sunday night and keep them in your refrigerator/freezer. This strategy can save you lots of time compared to preparing a fresh meal each night.

Thirdly, take a minute to reflect on your support system. To be successful at anything, having a strong and encouraging support system can help you reach your goals. You can ask your family and friends if they would like to diet with you, which can help make the process easier. If they do not want to diet with you, ask them to be supportive of your decision. You might even want to find somebody else who is dieting, eating healthy, or in being a workout buddy to help keep you motivated.

Fourthly, if you know you're going to eat out at a restaurant, try to find out what their menu is like beforehand. Make sure you take into account everything that you eat and try to pick out the healthiest options. You can even stick to your diet when eating out by making simple swaps, such as getting fresh vegetables instead of fries or skipping out on the free bread.

Fifthly, don't leave your sweet tooth in the dust. Being on a diet does not mean that you have to cut out tasty treats completely; it just means that you have to be more aware of what and how much you eat. If you tend to crave junk food, make room for it in your diet so that you don't binge on it later. A good idea is to set aside 100 calories in your diet for when you're having a junk food craving. Chocolate is always a favorite, and dark chocolate is actually healthy for you. Just choose something that you like as a reward for all your hard work

The best part about creating a personal diet plan is that you get to choose what kinds of foods you want to eat every day. As you begin to create your own diet plan, think about the different kinds of foods you can include from each food group. When planning out your meals, take these few tips into consideration:

You can stay full by combining protein and fiber. Your body will feel more satisfied from having a lunch that consists of a piece of fruit, a yogurt cup, and a cooked egg rather than a bag of chips and a soda. A really great, easy lunch that has worked out for me is combining four tablespoons of low-fat, vanilla yogurt with a bowl of pumpkin flavored granola. It keeps me full between breakfast and dinner and it's very healthy and tasty. I like vanilla and pumpkin flavors, but you can use any combination of yogurt and granola flavors to switch it up.

When going grocery shopping, try to opt for the low-fat options if they're available. For example, pick skim milk over whole milk and 93% ground beef over 73% ground beef. Also try to stick to natural foods instead of processed foods. For example, switching low-fat milk for whole milk can be effective because your body will still get calcium. You can also switch to Almond Milk, which is one of my favorites! It stays fresh for months at a time, tastes great, is healthy, and can be substituted for milk products quite easily.

Invest in a small kitchen scale and measuring cup set to help measure your meal proportions. Even though you can pretty much eat all the fruits and vegetables that you want without harming your body, it is easy to go overboard on things like cheese, meat, and pasta.

Chapter 9: Clean Eating

Clean eating is not a diet plan but rather a lifestyle. This is not something that you can follow just to lose weight and forego once you have achieved your weight loss goals. Eating clean is a practice that you and your family should ultimately live by for the rest of your lives.

The concept of clean eating has been practiced ever since the first man learned how to make use of the natural vegetation and wild animal resources in their areas. It is simply eating organic, lean and naturally obtained fruits, vegetables and meat using the simplest and the healthiest preparations.

To better understand what this healthy lifestyle is all about, you definitely need to find out more about its principles.

This is because you need to do some major changes in your life especially if you have been leading an unhealthy lifestyle by eating mostly junk foods, processed foods, or instant meals. Clean eating is not the same as those diet fads that promise to help you lose weight. This is more about improving the quality of food that you eat than limiting the quantity. It also has something to do with changing your eating habits and your lifestyle.

Most of the food items included in the clean eating diet plan are also recommended by public health groups and organizations. Compared to diet fads, clean eating is more flexible and can be adapted to almost all kinds of lifestyle.

To help you understand what clean eating is, you need to know the basic principles of clean eating.

Balance Diet is the Key.

Aim for the balanced diet for optimum health. This will encourage you to go for more balanced meals every single day. Whether you are snacking or having lunch, your plate should have the right proportions of carbs and protein. This will not only make your healthier, you will also be able to quell all your bouts of hunger and unrealistic cravings.

Explore your Kitchen

Home meals are better than foods prepared outside like fast foods. No matter how much these restaurants claim that they use nothing but the best products, you can never be too sure that they do not use processed food products. Clean eating will help you learn how to prepare fast, simple and healthy meals.

Processed Foods

Nowadays process foods are common practice to preserved foods and to make it lasts than it supposed to. Refined foods are processed foods that no longer have all the nutrients that they originally had. Certain foods have to undergo this process to improve their taste, give them a longer shelf life, and create a finer appearance and texture. One example is refined white sugar. It is best to choose unrefined brown sugar than white sugar for your coffee or tea. However, when it comes to baking, most recipes require the use of white sugar because it gives a smoother and silkier texture to the bread or pastry. But if you want to get the complete nutrients of the food, you have to make sure that you choose unrefined over refined food products

Prefer Whole Foods

Prefer whole unprocessed foods rather than processed ones. Canned, packed and labelled foods are considered to be processed types of food. The thing about such types of foods is that they may contain ingredients, such as preservatives that could be chemically laced and are harmful to your body. But if there are processed foods that you can eat, those would be whole grain pastas, vegan meat substitutes, organic grains and flours and cheeses. Every time you read the labels, keep in mind that if you cannot pronounce it, do not buy it!

Lesser sodium Intake.

The daily recommendation for sodium is only 2300 mg per day and most Americans eat 1,000 mg more sodium than the limit because they often eat fast foods and processed foods. To ensure that your sodium intake is still within the limit, you should consider eating out less frequently and cooking your own food at home. You can make your meals tastier even without adding too much salt by using spices and herbs.

Unprocessed Food

Unprocessed food are also known as whole foods which does not undergone any process and retain its original state. For example, whole grains are grains that still contain all the original layers or parts including the endosperm, germ, and bran. Grains that are crushed, cracked, or rolled are already considered processed. Natural foods are those that do not have any chemicals or artificial ingredients in them. Whole natural foods contain all the nutrients that are found in the original nutritional value of the food.

Meatless Diets

Meat is known to contain saturated fats that are bad for your health. However, you cannot completely eliminate meat from your diet because it is an important source of protein. What you can do is to use meat as flavouring to your meals instead of serving it as the meal itself. For example, instead of eating fried chicken for dinner, you should consider adding bits of chicken in your soup.

High Fibres

If there is one thing that cannot be overlooked in any diet plans is fibres rich foods. The best examples of these are fruits and vegetables. Everyone knows how beneficial fruits and vegetables are to your health. They contain vitamins and minerals that your body needs without having to worry about adding more calories. Fruits and vegetables also make you feel full longer, which prevents you from overeating. When choosing fruits and vegetables, be sure to pick those that came directly from the farm. You can buy fresh fruits and vegetables from your local farmer's market or stalls that sell produce.

Watch What You Drink

Some drinks are known to contain high caloric contents. Instead of drinking soft drinks or specialty coffees that are high in calories, you should consider drinking plain water instead. In the morning, you can drink low-fat skim milk, unsweetened tea, or freshly squeezed fruit juice for breakfast.

Eat Small Amount of Meals Frequently

Do not overeat at once. The clean eating diet plan encourages people to eat small meals about five to six times a day instead of eating two or three large meals. Skipping meals is not encouraged and eating healthy snacks in between meals is encouraged. This prevents you from overeating and keeps your energy level stable throughout the day.

The Reality of Saturated Fats

Contrary to popular belief, fats in general are not bad to your health. However, there is a specific kind of fats that you need to avoid called saturated fats. These fats are found in dairy products and meat. Clean eating does not mean that you should completely eliminate fats from your diet; in fact, that is not recommended because fats are also important to your health. What you need is to focus on good fats such as those found in canola oil, olive oil, nuts, and fish.

Moderate Alcohol Consumption

Everything in life should consume in moderation. You can still drink alcohol but you should limit your alcohol intake and avoid getting drunk. For women, the recommended limit for alcohol is one drink per day. For men, the limit is 2 drinks per day. Too much alcohol is bad for your health because it can cause dehydration and can add calories to your diet.

Watch your Sugar Intake

Sugar is the energy booster of the body but too much consumption of sugar can make your body to transform it into fats. Aside from sodium, you should also watch your sugar intake. The recommended sugar intake is 9 teaspoons for men and 6 teaspoons for women. You should avoid sugary foods like baked treats, candies, and soda. You should also watch out for healthy foods with added sugar like cereal, yogurt, and tomato sauce.

Chapter 10: Benefits of Clean Eating

Because of the kinds of food that you are encouraged to eat with the clean eating diet plan, you can get a lot of benefits that help improve your health. Some of the benefits of eating clean are listed in the paragraphs below.

Effectively Lose Weight

Foods promoted by clean eating diet makes your weight lose effectively. For instance, it promotes low sugar intake that helps you achieve optimum weight. It also encourages you to eat more fruits and vegetables and less meat which lowers your calorie intake. Aside from eating healthy foods, clean eating also promotes an active lifestyle. You can do some exercises or be more physically active that can help you lose weight.

Better Digestion

Consuming a lot of fast food often make our GI more acidic. Well, if you observe carefully, you will even hear your digestive enzymes struggle to work their way through all the oily processed foods that you have consumed. Clean eating will help put a stop to acid refluxes, indigestion and poor bowel movement. You will have all the fibre that you need to improve your digestion in so many ways.

Be a Chef of your Own

It is better to eat what you cook rather than eat what you do not see it coming. This lifestyle does not mean that you have to eat bland and dull looking meals every single time. Clean eating, with all the amazingly healthy ingredients that you can choose from, should and will encourage you to try new recipes to bring life to your dishes. Clean eating should get you excited to prepare your own meals!

Immunity Booster

Eating clean foods boost your immunity and also protects you against diseases like heart diseases, stroke, diabetes, and cancer. It helps lower your cholesterol level and boosts the strength of your blood vessels. Fruits and vegetables are also rich in vitamins and minerals that promote strong immunity that helps you fight illnesses. And because you are eating less saturated fat, the cholesterol level in your body is also regulated. The artificial and chemical ingredients in processed foods also increase risk of cancer. Fruits and vegetables are rich in antioxidants and phytonutrients that are known to help fight cancer cells.

Boost your Energy

In order to boost your energy you need to receive the right amount of vitamins and mineral needed for your body to function properly. For example, iron and vitamin B-complex improves cellular functions. Clean eating also promotes eating small meals more frequently. This helps regulate the sugar level in your blood stream which gives you a steady supply of energy throughout the day. This is also due to your reduced consumption of sweets and refined carbohydrates.

Improve you Mental Well Being

Aside from improving your physical health, eating clean foods also helps boost your mental health. Fish is rich in omega-3 fatty acids, a good kind of fat included in the clean eating diet plan. This fat helps fight depression and moodiness. Vitamin B-6, which can be found in sunflower seeds, pistachio nuts, and tuna, also helps produce dopamine, a hormone in the body that makes you feel good and happy.

Everyone's Diet

Many think that clean eating diet is only for those people who are health enthusiast and not applicable for everyone. Gone are the days when you think that healthy or clean eating is just for vegans, vegetarians, diabetes, heart patients or those who are on a really strict diet. Clean eating is for those who would like to take great care of themselves better.

Improves your Skin

What you eat reflects from the inside. If you are healthy from within, your outward appearance will also look healthy which includes your hair and skin. Some fruits and vegetables are rich in antioxidants that are known to fight wrinkles and skin blemishes. Fruits and vegetables also have higher water content, which keeps your skin hydrated at all times. You also do not have to worry about chemicals that can be harmful to your body and can cause damage to your skin.

Makes you More Satisfied in Eating

Clean eating diet makes you more satisfied when you eat. Unlike junk food makes you crave more food, which in turn makes you gain those unwanted pounds. Eating cleaner and healthier food will make sure that you will feel full and satisfied longer since you will be completely nourished.

Chapter 11 Clean Eating Tips That Will You Lose Weight Effectively

As stated clean eating is not a diet plan but rather a lifestyle modification. It is important that you know some useful tips that will help you lose weight and rejuvenate. You also need to know some tips on how to make clean and green eating a permanent part of your life. Remember that this is not just a diet fad that you only need to do for a limited timeframe. This requires significant changes in your routine and your life in general, which is why it is important that you plan the transition carefully. Here are some tips and ideas you might find useful.

Have an active lifestyle

Losing weight does not depend only in changing your diet alone. It is not enough to achieve your optimum weight and health. You also need to get the right amount of exercise that your body needs to burn the calories you get from the food you eat and prevent them from turning into fat. You need to exercise regularly if you want to lose weight and to keep yourself healthy. You can do some cardio workout and muscle and strength training that will help you lose weight and become more fit and healthy. You can either pay for a monthly gym membership where you have a personal trainer, or do the exercises yourself at the park or at home.

Aside from regular workouts, you can also get enough exercise by being more physically active. Instead of driving your car to buy a carton of milk at the grocery just a couple of blocks away from your house, you should consider walking or riding your bike. Instead of using the elevator, you can use the stairs to go to your office floor, unless of course your office is located on the 23rd floor or something. If that's the case, you should consider riding the elevator halfway or two-thirds up then using the stairs for the remaining few floors.

Spices

Spices and herbs are excellent addition to your dishes. But if you are a bit scared to try new spices and seasoning blends, why don't you go for herbs and other ingredients that could elevate and take your healthy meals to whole new levels? Try experimenting and incorporating these healthy herbs and spices in your next recipes:

Sleep

Sleep helps you to rejuvenate and boost your body for the strenuous activities for the day. This will allow you to perform your tasks more efficiently. It is also easier to follow your clean eating lifestyle if you have enough energy. For example, you will have the energy to prepare clean meals throughout the day and do some exercises if your body is well-rested.

Meal Plans

Planning your meals helps you to get the necessary discipline for proper dieting. Make the internet your best friend, or this book to look for amazingly delicious but unbelievably healthy dishes that you can easily make for your family. You can create a chart and plan what you will be cooking and eating for a week or in the next few days.

Food Pyramid

Clean eating strongly advocates balanced eating. Eating whole, natural foods will be useless if you do not get the recommended amount of all the food groups. You need to know what foods are great sources of protein, carbohydrates, good fats, vitamins, minerals, fibre, and other nutrients that your body needs. It is important to get the recommended amount of each of these nutrients in your diet because they have different functions that keep you healthy and improve your general well-being. For instance, fibber's main function is to flush out toxins in your body and improve your bowel movement. Protein, on the other hand, improves your strength and muscles.

Be Master of your Own Kitchen

Learn to explore your Kitchen. Do not be afraid to get out of your comfort zone and experiment on different healthy recipes that you have found. You can try small portions first and see if you and the rest of the family will like what you have prepared.

Nutrition Facts

Many of us simply eat without reading the nutrional facts. Any health conscious individual should know how to read nutrition labels because this is where you can find the amount of nutrients that the food item contains. The nutrition label usually includes macronutrients such as protein, carbohydrates, and fats. It also includes vitamins and minerals. You will also know the calories that the food product has and the number of servings per package. It is important that you know how to read nutrition labels to ensure that you are getting the adequate amount of required nutrients.

Aside from the nutrition label, you also need to know how to read the ingredients list. One useful tip is to avoid any food item that has an ingredient whose name is too long and difficult to pronounce because it is most likely an artificial or chemical ingredient.

Prepare foods ahead of time

Learn to prepare food ahead of time to save time and effort. You really do not have to be a slave in the kitchen every day, because there are healthy or nutritious meals that you can make ahead of time, store in the fridge and reheat. You can even label the containers with the dates or day that they should be consumed to keep their freshness and maintain their flavours.

Good Living

Aim for clean living. Clean eating does not completely forbid you to drink alcohol but there is a recommended amount which is 1 drink for women and 2 drinks for men. You should also quit smoking and stop using illegal drugs if you want to stay healthy, lose weight, and make clean eating a permanent part of your life. Aside from these, you also need to stop doing bad habits like staying up really late at night, skipping meals, and eating fast food and takeout all the time.

Shopping List

Prepare a shopping list for convenience and to prevent over buying. Do not get too overly excited to shop for fruits, veggies, meats and dairy products. Keep a record of what ingredients you have and take note of their expiration dates; this list will serve are your reference for the next time that you will go grocery shopping.

Use your Fridge

Check your fridge for a possible stock up. Another important tip to adapt a clean eating habit is to stock up on clean foods like fresh fruits and vegetables, whole bread and pasta, lean meat, skinless poultry, and so on. It will be easier to follow your clean eating diet if you already have something to cook in your kitchen. Most of the time, people go back to their old eating habits because they do not have something to cook in their kitchen. Buying clean foods is not difficult because you can easily find them in your local grocery or market. You need to prepare a 7-day meal plan at the start of the week so that you will know what you need to buy when you go grocery shopping. This will prevent you from going back to your old ways because you already have your meals and grocery shopping planned.

Cooking can be Fun

Cooking can be fun if you learn it and enjoy it. It is also easier to follow the clean eating lifestyle if you know how to cook. There may be some restaurants that offer clean foods but they can be difficult to find. If you know how to cook, you do not have to worry about finding the right restaurant that uses clean foods for their meals. Cooking your own food also gives variety. You will get tired of eating the same foods from the local restaurant that offers clean foods in your area. You do not have to be a chef to prepare clean meals. You can use simple recipes at first before moving on to more difficult and elaborate recipes

Chapter 12: Natural Ways to Get Fit

There are many natural ways to get fit. In order to achieve a physical fit body you need to condition your mind to have a more proper mindset. Everything starts on how you view things and how motivated you are to achieve it. Learning the proper ways to balance your mind and your lifestyle is an essential part in achieving fit and healthy body.

Take Charge of Your Mind

Taking charge of what you think takes enough discipline and focus and it is necessary in achieving fitness as whole. This can only be achieve by means of meditation. Meditation is a state of thoughtless awareness. It is not about effort or doing, rather it is simply a state of awareness.

According to Indian mystic, guru and spiritual teacher, Osho "All that the mind is capable of doing and achieving is not relevant when it comes to meditation – meditation is something beyond the mind. The mind is absolutely helpless when it comes to meditation."

Osho goes on to say that "The mind cannot penetrate meditation; where mind ends, meditation begins."

You and I have been taught to believe that everything can be done with the mind. So, when it comes to meditation, our natural inclination is to start thinking in terms of techniques, methods and what we can do to maximize our meditational experience.

It makes sense that we would think this way because so many things in life validate the use of the mind in getting what we want. We have been raised with the belief that "if you just put your mind to it, you can do anything." There is truth to that, yet the only thing that the mind cannot "do" is meditate.

Meditation techniques will teach you how to take control of and connect with your mind, but the necessity of that control only pertains to the degree in which it allows you to free yourself from your mind.

Meditation is your true nature. It is your being. It is fully you and it can only be entered into through the emptying of your mind. As Osho teaches "Meditation is not an achievement – it is something that already exists in you, it is your nature. It is there waiting for you – just turn inward and it is available. You have been carrying it always."

Meditation therefore is the simple process of removing your attention from current conditions and circumstances which when focused on too regularly fragment and cloud your perceptions.

When you allow for clear, unadulterated levels of conscious awareness to occur you access the spiritual being inside of you. This Spirit being is superior to your human mind and physical body and offers guidance and peace that you are unable to achieve at a human level.

As you consistently and patiently learn how to empty your mind, the deepened focus and concentration that you immerse yourself in will slowly create in you an intensely peaceful, powerful, clear and energized state of mind.

This spiritually energized state of mind is your intrinsic, Spirit nature that can guide and lead you in Truth and cause a transformative effect that will give you a new understanding of life.

What you can get in Meditation

As meditation increased in popularity over the years, more and more studies were conducted to explore the effects of meditation on the human mind and body. Scientists extensively researched the potential benefits of meditation and how it could help cure a wide range of physical, mental, emotional and even societal ailments.

Since its introduction in 1959, more than 600 research studies on meditation were carried out at 250 different universities and medical schools around the world to confirm the effectiveness of meditation.

The National Institutes of Health in the United States granted more than $24 million for research studies on the topic of meditation. These research studies are now recorded in more than 650 scientific and medical journals each of which provide proof of the benefits of meditation for medical conditions such as diabetes, cancer, chronic pain and heart disease.

Because of the deemed benefits of meditation, many businesses have started sponsoring meditation classes for their employees' well-being. This cost-effective solution enhances employee productivity and keeps employees happy.

Even public schools in the United States have started to teach meditation to both children and teenagers. Research study conducted by the Medical College of Georgia in 2003 discovered that meditation lowers stress and enhances interpersonal relationships between students. It was also discovered that it improves school performance.

The government has also started using meditation to lower crime rates and the US military uses meditation as an effective treatment for post-traumatic stress disorder acquired by soldiers sent out to war.

Meditation has been practiced in the East for several centuries though it is fairly new to the western world. Its benefits and ease of implementation has been easily recognized by western culture which has led to its rapid popularity growth.

For just a few minutes a day, with absolutely no cost or special equipment, anyone can take advantage of the benefits of meditation.

Despite its simplicity, the overall efficacy of meditation has made it the most valuable means for people to heal not only themselves but the planet as well.

Reduces inflammation –Stress leads to inflammation. Relaxation turns off the stress response therefore reducing the health risks caused by inflammation

Lowers high blood pressure by making the body less responsive to stress hormones

Decreases anxiety attacks by lowering the levels of blood lactate

Boosts the production of serotonin that improves mood and behavior

Reduces stress-related ailments including headaches, insomnia and ulcers

Boosts the immune system

Improves energy levels

Balance Your Energy

Regulating your food input is one of the natural way to balance your weight. Managing your mind on what food to eat creating discipline and well manage diet. Calories are the measurement units of energy balance. They measure the potential heat energy in the food and drink we consume. Calories represent fuel that the body needs to function.

Daily food intake is the consumption of calories. Daily activities and the body's basic physiological tasks expend or use calories.

The human body functions on a supply and demand system. If the daily consumption of calories meets the body's demand--the excess calories are stored for future use, in the form of fat. The reserves of stored fat are available for energy usage when the body's demand for calories exceeds the daily calorie consumption.

3,500 calories is equal to one pound. If you consume 3,500 more calories than you burn over a period of time—you will gain one pound. If you consumer 3,500 less calories than you burn over a period of time—you will lose one pound.

Your weight and management of your weight is dependent upon this one simple principle.

Be the Pilot of Your Own Fitness

Taking charge of your own body is an integral part of achieving fitness. Do not simply rely on others or guided diet plans to lose weight but takes an active part in making things work for you. Some people form a habit in blaming everything to others on the things they cannot take accountabilities of themselves. Here are some checklist you can take note on.

Be honest on yourself

Be honest with yourself that is the key. Taking charge starts with taking stock of yourself and your unique and current situation. This must be an honest and thorough personal assessment, but without any judgment. You simply want to be objective and accurate about where you are from a fitness perspective--so that you can develop the right knowledge, goals, mental programming, and action plan for long-term success.

What is going on in your life that affects your fitness and weight? How does your body really look? Be honest about your body. At this point, what goals can realistically be set to move you toward fitness and your target weight?

Gaining a deeper understanding of your motivation, fears, strengths, weaknesses, and unique fitness personality is a proven and effective strategy for developing a plan that will inspire you to stick with it—develop the fitness habit—and maintain a fitness lifestyle.

Take the Moment

We've all had moments in our lives when we are excited about something new—a change or an up-coming event. Yet, at the same time--we are filled with anxiety, doubt, and maybe even fear--because we are not certain of how or where to begin.

Sometimes, we are not sure how to get started with our fitness program. In that precise moment of uncertainty or indecision--you can either allow the excitement to propel you forward, or you can concede and allow the "status quo" of not taking action to continue.

The daily moments of key decision-making are crucial to your fitness motivation and success. You must acknowledge the power of these "daily decision points" as they are truly defining moments. The daily decision points are a gift and opportunity to move forward toward your improved fitness--or they can be an excuse to slide backward toward being more overweight and unhealthy.

It's your choice. You have the power! Seize the opportunity to take charge of your fitness and health by simply making your daily decision points work for you and not against you.

Be Responsible Enough

Taking responsibility on your own fitness is the stepping stone in any fitness regimen. When you take charge and accept full responsibility for your fitness without excuses—you will be more self-directed, self-reliant, and consistent in your actions and achievements. Assuming full responsibility for your fitness motivation will help you maintain your fitness motivation.

I encourage you to enlist others to help you. Positive and knowledgeable supporters can contribute tremendously to your motivation, fitness success, and weight loss accomplishments. However, you must ultimately play the central role in your own fitness and weight loss success.

Be bold and proud in assuming full responsibility for all of your results as you start your fitness program. Don't be afraid to share your successes and failures with your core supporters. You will often gain insights and inspiration from others.

Use your growing knowledge and confidence to assess results constantly, so that you can quickly correct mistakes. The motivating power of consistent improvement and results will eventually override and eliminate fear if you are willing to take full responsibility for your success!

Chapter 13: Take a Walk

Walking is the most natural way to lose weight. Walking is easy. Most of us do it every day, sometimes without even thinking about it. If you are fortunate not to have any health problems, you may find yourself as a busy professional who knows the quickest route to drive somewhere, and always looks for the first row parking spot. Can you walk? Yes, but you don't have time. You are a professional, and you have responsibilities.

If you are retired, you work from home, or if you are a stay at home parent, you may find that you have time to walk on some days, but don't have time to walk on other days. It's hard to know what your day is going to look like when it begins, and sometimes you are hesitant to commit to anything that you know you won't be able to keep up. You don't have a gym membership, you don't make plans more than one day out, or maybe you find joy and freedom in making plans impulsively.

Maybe you just have low-self-esteem right now. Maybe you're grieving, maybe you're at a rough patch in your life, maybe you're unemployed, or you're a little more overweight than you thought you were. Maybe you realize that a change needs to happen, but you're so comfortable in the life you have that you're afraid of being shot down again. You don't have the energy to try something new. You want change, but you don't know how to make it.

Would you believe that walking will boost your confidence, irrespective of whatever lifestyle you adopt?

Why do you think that elementary school students have recess every day? Yes, on the surface it's because they're highly energetic children who need time to run around and get a little tired so that they can sit in their chairs again, but any teacher will tell you that even the best students learn better if they get up and move around between long periods of study.

Let's take this concept to adults: you could be a professional, but that doesn't mean that you're confident —and you may very well be confident, but it's likely that being a professional means that you're stressed out about work often as well.

By getting into the habit of going for a walk every day at a time of your choosing (most professionals enjoy a walk first thing in the morning, but based on your work or what time you get off you may find that walking when you get home at the end of the day is suitable as well) will relax you and ground you more.

By managing something easy like walking, you are in control, you are responsible, and you are taking initiative to do something good for yourself. That's confidence.

If you're retired, work from home, or a stay at home parent, this concept is no different. Sometimes you don't know what your day is going to be like because you a lot of other factors monopolize your schedule.

If you commit to walking daily or every other day in a block of time that is untouched by other things, you will find yourself more confident because you are in control of something. This doesn't mean that the other things in your life are bad or that they need to stop. However, by adding something for you and only for you that you can control will breed confidence.

If you are going through a rough patch in your life and you know you need to make a change but don't know what it is, go for a walk around the block. The fresh air will be good, the circulation will be good, and you don't have to be gone a long time. Fresh air is the lifeblood of circulation, and circulation helps things to move. In your case, they could move you from this place you find yourself in.

Confidence is having control, and walking is an easily controlled, healthy activity. You can walk around the block or you can walk a 3 mile hiking trail—it doesn't matter. You are in control; it is up to you how, where, and for how long you want to walk.

What is an area of your schedule that you can control? You don't have to commit to it yet, just jot a few ideas down in a journal. Next, write about how you would feel if you have one small area of your life that you could control, and how you would feel if this small thing could also provide health benefits, make you feel better, and potentially help you lose weight.

Right Tools for Walking

If you decide to take walking seriously you need to wear the right shoes to achieve the fitness you want to achieve. If you select shoes that do not fit correctly, that hurt your feet or are not flexible enough, you will learn to hate your walking experience.

You will have to end up deciding which shoe will be best for you, although there are a few simple things you should take into consideration when making your choice.

All about shoes

If you take walking seriously see to it that you are choosing the correct size shoe. You do not want your foot sliding around in a shoe that is far too big. On the opposite end of the equation, you do not want your toes cramped up in the front of the shoe. Even walking for five minutes with shoes like these can cause damage to your feet.

You will have a fair idea of your correct shoe size. Of course, all manufacturers are different, so be sure to try the shoes on, and perhaps more importantly, walk a fair distance in both of them. If you feel any form of discomfort, try another pair.

Walk down an incline as well as upstairs when trying out the shoes. When walking down an incline, your toes should not move forward at all, and should never touch the front of the shoe. Walking on stairs helps to gauge how much your heels will lift when going uphill. Consider trying a new pair of shoes if your heel moves more than 0.3 centimeters. This indicates that you may suffer from blistering to your heel.

Ideally, there should be around a centimeter between where the toes end and the front of the shoe, allowing for some movement for your foot, very important when travelling down steep gradients. Remember to check the width of the shoe as well. Your toes should be spaciously spread out and not crumpled together because the shoe is not wide enough.

When buying a new pair of walking shoes, it is best to try them on at the end of a long day. At this point your feet will be swollen from your day's activities. Try to take a pair of socks with that you will use during walking, or at least the same kind of thickness.

The shoes that you choose should be fairly flexible. Take then in your hands and twist. Do they bend and flex easily? A good walking shoe should!

Why does a shoe need to be flexible? At the end of the day, it all comes down to comfort. As you take each step, your foot flexes as first the heel, then the middle and finally your toes strike the surface. Your shoe therefore should do the same. If not, the natural motion your foot makes when striking the ground will work against the inflexible shoe and this can lead to shin splints.

Perform this quick check. Take the shoe and twist it. It should twist very easily and come back to its proper shape. Then bend the shoe. Make sure it bends where the ball of your foot would be and not around the middle section of the arch. Finally, place the shoe on the ground and push down on where your front toe would be. Does the shoe rock slightly? If so, then the shoe passes the flexibility test.

Also check to see that the material the shoe is made out of will be able to breathe efficiently, allowing sweat from your feet the chance to evaporate effectively.

As you will be walking fair distances in your shoes, you should ensure that they have the correct cushioning to protect your feet. Luckily, a walking shoe does not require as much cushioning as a running shoe might, but it should still have enough support. The most important areas for cushioning are the heel as well as the ball of the foot as these are first to strike the ground.

There are a number of minor factors that you can also consider when purchasing your walking shoes.

- The lighter the shoes the better, especially if you are walking a fair distance.
- Some form of shock absorption (especially in the cushioning), can make the shoes more comfortable.
- Depending on weather conditions in the area that you walk, you may consider buying a shoe that is waterproof.
- Pick shoes with low heels that provide support. Thicker, wider heels often cause the feet to hit the tarmac very hard instead of falling in a nice rolling motion. This results in a loss of momentum and increased irritation on the shins.
- Always try to walk your shoes in by wearing them for a few days around the house before using them for a walking workout.

Although not as important as choosing the correct shoes, there are a number of clothing items that you can consider to enhance your walking experience.

When choosing the correct clothing, these are the aspects you should take into account:

- Socks.

- Clothing for specific weather conditions.
- Accessories

Socks

Choosing the right socks is as important as choosing the right shoes. Socks need to do a number of things. Firstly, they offer a second barrier of protection to your feet after your shoes. Secondly, the sock must be able to allow any perspiration from your feet to evaporate properly. If they are unable to do this, walking will not only be uncomfortable, possibly leading to blisters, but your shoes will end up damaged.

The best socks in this regards are made out of an all-synthetic material. If you go on long walks and suffer with very sweaty feet, you may consider changing your socks fairly often, but especially if they are wet with perspiration.

Socks can also offer padding around the heel and ball of the foot, providing even more comfort.

Clothes

Clothes is an essential considerations in walking regimen. And walking in different weather conditions needs special considerations.

When walking in hot weather, try to wear synthetic fibers that do not absorb sweat. Always aim to wear fairly light colors as these will help to reflect both the light and heat of the sun, leaving you cooler. Wear a hat to prevent sunburn and dehydration.

In cold weather, it is critical to wear layers of clothing to keep the warmth in. Pay particular attention to your exposed body parts such as your hands. The first layer of clothing should be synthetic material to allow any perspiration to evaporate. A second layer should be insulating, helping to ensure that body heat is trapped in. These layers can be wool or light fleece. A zipper on this layer can help control the levels of heat. The third layer is often the outer layer, and should not only be water resistant, but also have the ability to keep the wind out.

Accessories

Wearing accessories can help you to make your walking much better. There are numerous accessories that you can use while walking.

- Sunglasses. These are very important for protecting your eyes, especially in sunny conditions.
- Water bottle/CamelBak. Even if you are only walking for twenty minutes, water is essential to keep you hydrated. For longer walks try to drink water at least every 20 minutes.
- Heart rate monitor. A heart rate monitor can be particularly useful if you are want to keep your heart rate at a constant level, especially when trying to keep a fat burning zone.
- Pedometer. A pedometer is a great little gadget that helps to count all the steps you have made. You should be aiming to build up to around 10 000 steps a day.
- Music. A lot of walkers enjoy the accompaniment of music. You may consider a personal music device to help make the miles fly by!

Benefits

Walking is definitely one of best way of losing weight. Walking is not a very vigorous way to lose weight as going to a gym is, but it is very effective nevertheless. You can safely say that walking is one of the most ancient exercises and still one of the best that are practiced.

But the fact about walking is you can lethargically take a walk in the park and expect to lose weight. Your weight loss depends on its intensity and continuity. You should walk regularly to see positive results in terms of weight loss. The progress may be slow and steady, but in the long run it is extremely effective.

If you intend to lose the flab on your body and are confused which exercise regimen works best for you, then the best option is to start with walking. Don't even give it a second thought; just take up regular walking. The best part about walking is that it can be practiced by any age group. Whether you are 15 or 80, you can choose walking as a fitness option.

There are a number of health advantages to walking regularly.

On the surface, it seems that the only benefits are control, confidence, and peace of mind. These are very strong and important benefits (and later we'll see why these are more important than we think they are). If you have control, confidence, and peace of mind, walking helps to improve your daily life. The rest of your personal or professional schedule may not change, but at least if you have control over one activity that is just yours, you may find that you have peace of mind over those other daily duties.

It's often recommended that widows or widowers get a dog after a spouse has passed away. While it seems like a difficult responsibility to take care of something else when you need taking care of yourself, physicians have found that widows and widowers who follow this instruction are less despondent not only because he or she is taking care of something that will love him/her unconditionally, but also the widow or widower now has the responsibility of taking that dog for daily or twice-daily walks.

Walking the dog gets the bereaved spouse out of the house, out into fresh air, meeting neighbors, having companionship, and controlling at least one small aspect of his or her life.

Your mindset is everything to your health. Once you start recognizing confidence, responsibility, and peace of mind over this easy, small thing that you can control, physicians have found that walkers have lower blood pressure. Why? To some, it's because stress has been reduced through an outlet. To others it's an exercise. However, walking provides peace of mind to everyone who practices it.

Other health benefits of walking regularly include muscle toning. Because you're walking at a regular, slower pace than, say, jogging, you have the flexibility to work with different muscle groups. Some walkers will walk on their toes for a brief while to stretch out their hamstrings, some walkers bend their knees more to work out their calves more, some walkers take extra-large steps occasionally as if lunging, and some walkers will start out at a slow pace, escalate to a fast pace, and then decelerate back to a slow pace before arriving at his or her home.

But whether you actively work on muscle toning or not, walking regularly is an effective aid to weight loss. In recent years, doctors have found that more patients who walk regularly lose more weight than patients who jog. The reason for this is because walking is gentler on your system (particularly on your joints, your skeletal system, and your back) so walkers have the ability to walk longer more regularly than joggers who might take the day off because of joint pain. Walkers generally have more endurance than some joggers and stay active and healthy longer into their life than joggers who quit when they get "too old" or have too many extenuating circumstances. Walking is easy, and for some it's easy to commit to daily or every other day.

Walking is the safest form of exercise, so it is ideal for everyone no matter what body type or age they are. While walking doesn't cause weight loss overnight, if you walk 15-20 minutes 3-5 times a week, you'll lose about half a pound to a pound a week. While this doesn't sound like a lot, keeping this regimen up for 20 weeks results in weight loss up to 20 lbs.

The average amount of weight loss per person varies for however many minutes they walk. However, the more you weigh the more calories you burn during a 15-20 minute walk. This is particularly beneficial for those who might think they're too overweight to start a workout regimen: the heavier you are, the more walking will help you lose weight. The more weight you lose, the more confident you will feel, and the healthier you will be.

- Walking is one of the best exercises to get back in shape.
- It increases your metabolism; thereby your body burns more calories.
- Walking when practiced regularly, helps keep many illnesses at bay
- Individuals who suffer from bone and joint related diseases like, osteoarthritis, osteoporosis get relief with regular walking.
- Walking decreases the tension in your bones, making the bones stronger.
- Walking outside during daytime provides you with vitamin D, which is very important for your bones to be strong and healthy.
- It helps in maintaining healthy joints.
- Walking helps you to tackle diseases like hypertension and diabetes.
- Regular walking practice for 30 minutes or more helps improve the blood glucose level and heart rate.
- When you walk your elbows are bent and your hands swing back and forth. This continuous motion helps you to get rid of extra baby fat from your arms.
- Walking also works on your lower body. It helps you tone your hamstrings, thighs and also the gluteal region.
- Walking shapes your legs, and gives a great definition to the calves.

- Walking helps relieves mental stress and relaxes your mind.
- It makes you feel fresh, and revives your mind.
- You tend to make new friends while walking (or spend time with a walking buddy), so your social life improves.
- Walking leads to weight loss. When you see positive results, it helps build self-confidence and a feeling of positivity

There are very few people who will randomly pick up a book on walking and decide that this is going to be their nightly reading material. Instead, most of the readers of this book are here with a struggle or a problem on their hands and they're looking for the first step to resolving that problem. Regardless of why you're here, most of those problems can be shaded by the umbrella of wanting a healthier life. So, what does that entail exactly?

By walking, you are fundamentally awakening your body out of a sense of dormancy. Walking is a full body workout. Not only are you testing the endurance of the muscles that you have, but you're also forcing your body weight to be carried by your legs which in turn form a light weight training exercise. You'll feel it in your legs most of all and that's a good thing. Walking is going to be your body's first contact with a healthier you and I guarantee you, you're going to feel it.

People who have never gone on a long walk will be very surprised about how much pain they're in the following morning. Now, mind you, this isn't a dreadful or agonizing pain. If it feels like something more than an ache in your muscles, then you need to consult a doctor right away. In fact, if there is any sharp, stabbing, or knife like pain in any part of your legs after walking, you should really consult your doctor immediately. Most likely, he will encourage you to get a wrap or brace for you knee or ankle.

You will, however, feel a definite ache in your legs and that's a really, really good thing for you to experience. That's the feeling of your muscle breaking down and needing to rebuild itself. That's the core of exercise. You are doing routines that break down a pre-existing muscle. This, in turn, tells your body that it needs to reinforce this damaged muscle and build it stronger. Your body then starts delegating nutrients and proteins to be redirected to the damaged muscle. Thus, your muscles are rebuilt stronger, tougher, and healthier.

In order to start working out and seeing the best possible progress, there are some dietary changes that you should start changing or incorporating. First of all, start drinking more water. The truth is, we could all do with a little more water in our lives and that means that we're more hydrated, more prepared, and healthier all over. So start drinking more water. Take a water bottle with you when you're walking. It'll help keep you hydrated and let you go on longer walks. Secondly, start taking a multivitamin. These are simple to get a hold of at any supermarket that you frequent. This will help make sure that the right vitamins and minerals that you're not getting in your diet is getting distributed to your injured muscle. Finally, start eating healthier. Have a salad, eat more vegetables, incorporate more fruit, and eat meat that isn't deep-fried. All of these will help you rebuild the muscles to the best of their ability and you'll see better results further on down the line.

These are all ways to help you incorporate a healthier way of living into your life and make you see the results that you're looking for. Now, let's have a look at where you should start when you decide to take up walking.

Chapter 14: Run for Your Life

Running is the most natural way to lose weight. Running is also an excellent way to experience the joys of life and reduce its pain and sorrows. I can attest to that. Whenever I encounter challenges that seem to be too big for me at the moment, I run. Not away from it, mind you but around the village in order to release all my pent up stress energy, which allows me to relax and put my mind in the best possible condition to either solve the problem or figure out the next steps toward it. Often times, nervous tension energy distracts us too much to concentrate on solving a problem and when we run, we release much of that energy to help calm us down and focus.

Another reason why we were born to run is to live. In fact, our primitive ancestors couldn't have survived much if they didn't know how to run. Can you imagine surviving in the wild, where savage beasts abound, simply by brisk walking yourself to safety when pursued by such? Unless those beasts are very poor brisk walkers, your chances of surviving are as high as skinny models' chances of going for seconds on a buffet party.

Aside from surviving ferocious animal attacks, our primitive ancestors also ran in order to hunt for food. Think about this, primitive men weren't born with spears in their hands, right? Given that, how'd you think they hunted for food? Well, they were born with feet, which they used for what is called persistence hunting.

Persistence hunting is a way of hunting animals by tracking them continuously by running and walking until they are exhausted enough to be, you know, hunted. You may be wondering, aren't most animals much faster runners than us humans? You are right in such wondering, my friend. What most people don't know however is that humans are built for endurance running and most animals aren't?

But what made it possible for our ancestors to engage in persistence hunting for survival? One word: sweat!

Runners Body Composition

No amount of glycogen stores and cooling system would be enough to make us born to run. What's possibly more important is our physiological structure. Look, snakes have a very efficient cooling system – they're cold-blooded for crying out loud! But do they have the body parts to run? I say no.

What makes us humans stand out from other mammals that run the earth are the spring like ligaments and tendons in the feet, butt muscles and our big toe. Let's take a closer look at why these conspire to make us natural born runners.

Tendons and ligaments in our feet and help us run efficiently because these parts make it possible for the body to absorb impact and propel the body much like what springs and shock absorbers do. Let's face it, running is an impact activity, i.e., subjects the body to impact when feet hit the pavement. Tendons and ligaments help absorb much of that impact and store the energy produced by it and release it to propel us forward. To further illustrate the point, have you ever tried running with your foot locked straight? Now you have an idea of the why tendons and ligaments help absorb impact and the resulting energy as well as to release such energy for propulsion.

But wait, there's more! Pardon the pun but yes, our butts are another reason why we're much better runners than animals. To be able to run quite a distance, we also need to stabilize our trunks...and I am not talking' about Speedos here. Butt muscles – better known as glutes (short for its scientific name gluteus maximus and minimums) – attach the hip to the base of the spine, making it possible for us to run with great stability. Glutes also make us look good in tucked in pants! Don't believe me? Check out a chimpanzee in pants and see how hip-foppish that looks!

The big toe is also a big difference maker when it comes to running. Being the last body part to leave the ground when running, it's the main body part used for pushing off the body much like the fingertips are the ultimate follow-through instruments when shooting a basketball. What makes the big toe such a big difference maker is the fact that unlike the big toes of apes and other non-running related species, ours is pretty much lined up with the other toes. In layman's terms, this lined-up position makes for a great running advantage.

Cry Your Skin Out

Have you ever seen your pet dogs or cats sweat? Have you ever seen horses sweat? Have you ever seen fish sweat? I'd bet your answer is no. This doesn't mean that they don't sweat, save probably for your goldfish. It only means they don't have the ability to sweat as much as we can.

Take for example your pet dog or cat. Their sweating is concentrated primarily on their faces (particularly the nose and mouth) and paws. They don't sweat anywhere else. This is why you notice that their noses and mouths are usually wet, especially on hot days. Horses and cows also don't sweat as much as you do on a hot and humid day. What this means is that their cooling mechanisms aren't anywhere near as efficient as people's and as such, makes them susceptible to overheating and exhaustion much quicker than we do – 10 to 15 minutes on average. Because they overheat faster, our ancestors were eventually able to subdue and, yum, eat them.

Have you ever tried taking your dog out for a run, especially on a hot and humid day? Do your dog a favor and just go for a walk with him or her because they won't be able to keep up. Their cooling systems aren't anywhere near yours or mine.

Sugar

Sugar or simple glucose is an energy fuel of our cells. Glucose is what becomes of the carbohydrates we consume. Think of the liver as the body's fuel tank. When you exercise in the morning before eating breakfast, this is the primary fuel your muscles use.

It is believed that most humans' livers contain on average 20 miles' worth of glycogen. That's quite a long run, if you ask me. Just like a high-performance sports car relies on a very efficient cooling system and the best fuels to go far and fast, so does the human body. Our bodies' ability to store much more glycogen than most other animals combined with a much better cooling system (sweat) allowed our ancestors to survive via persistence hunting. It also makes us natural born runners.

Benefits

Running reaps more benefits than you can imagine. People who take up running do it to either lose weight or to stay healthy. Running is the best form of exercise especially for people who want to reduce a few pounds without hitting the gym. It doesn't just provide good exercise for your body; it also helps in increasing stamina. Here are a few more reasons why running is beneficial.

- The first and foremost reason to take up running is the fact that it helps you burn calories faster and in a healthy manner.

If you are the outdoorsy types, this is by far the best exercise that will help you burn the fat.

- The feeling of exhilaration and high that you get from running are well worth the time and effort you make to run. It also boosts the serotonin levels in your brain and helps you relax and calms your mind. It's a great stress buster and good for your overall mental wellness.
- One of the best and prolonged effects of running is strong lungs. As compared to most of types of exercising, running improves your lung capacity.
- Stop the Blood pressure pills and wear your running shoes. Regular running expand and contract your arteries, which helps in regulating your BP
- When you run for a long time, it puts stress on your bones. When your bones are put under stress, your body sends out essential minerals, which in turn make them strong and improves their density. Not to forget the fact that you also get strong legs when you run regularly.
- You don't need to pay anyone. You don't need any special gadgets, machines or training. All you have to do is put your right foot forward then your left foot forward and repeat this process till whatever time you want.
- You can run in the park, in a field, on a track, on a hill, anywhere you want to run, you are free to do it. Then there is the good old treadmill if you are not particularly fond of the outdoors. As long as you have the will to run, you have a way to do it.
- Various studies have found that the calorie burning effects of exercises like running, which have a high intensity, stay for a longer time when you've stopped the exercise as compared to the exercises that are of a lower intensity, example: walking.
- You burn more calories while running than you would if you were walking or doing an exercise of a lower intensity in the same amount of time.

Running and Weight Loss

You may have heard this many times, but let me educate you again, weight loss is not all about exercise; you need to watch what you eat too. So if you want to get the maximum benefits from running, you need to focus on your diet too. Maintain a food dairy wherein you record the details of what you eat, how much you eat and the calorie content of that food. Plan your meals a day earlier, just as you plan your running (time, distance etc.). Eat right and take good care of yourself.

Instead of a slow, steady and long run all the time, run at a slow pace for about a minute and then increase the intensity for about half a minute. Repeat this many times during your run. This way, fat loss will be increased.

If you are running on a flat road or ground, try running on some inclined area or hill. You will burn more calories and lose more fat. Run up the incline for a few seconds, rest a few seconds and jog back. If you have no hill in your vicinity, then you can use the treadmill for this purpose at a 5% incline for a few seconds. Then set it back to normal for some time. Repeat it a few times.

Run upstairs and return back jogging slowly. This helps in fat loss.

Mostly runners run about twice a week or a maximum of 4 times a week. This is not sufficient for fat loss or weight loss. If you run more often, your metabolic activity is increased and you burn more calories results in more fat loss. You will also be a better runner this way. Fat loss should be gradual. This helps you perform better.

If you are a new runner, then start with short runs. Increase gradually the distance as well as intensity. Start off your eating for weight loss simultaneously by first stopping all the extra calories you are consuming. Start having nutritious food to improve your health. Reduce the quantity of the food you have been eating until now.

Replace all the junk food or high calorie food with nutritious and lower calorie foods.

For experienced runners, it is not possible to lose weight by increasing their intensity slowly as they are already into intense training. They can increase their running by 4-5 miles per session. It might help them to lose weight.

Body composition of regular runners can be improved through diet. Runners have to reduce the amount of fat in their diet in order to lose weight and improve the body composition. Fat helps gain weight in runners so cut down on fats. This in turn makes you lean. Every gram of fat has more than twice the amount of calories that is present in a gram of carbohydrate or protein.

Fat is absorbed faster as compared to proteins or carbohydrates. Lesser energy is spent to process fat. Weight loss takes places only when the daily intake reduces. So in other words if you as a runner reduce or remove rich fat food from your daily diet, the calories are automatically reduced and you have high chances of losing weight. You can replace the rich fats with low fat products which have lesser calories.

Remember not to eliminate it totally. Only reduce it. If you eliminate it totally, you will end up with vitamin and mineral deficiencies. Try to have monounsaturated fats and omega -3 fats as much as possible. So if you plan your diet carefully, weight loss can take place.

At times people want rapid weight loss and end up eating about 900-1000 calories on a daily basis. Since you will be reducing your total calorie intake, naturally your carbohydrate intake will also be low. Because of this the glycogen stored in the muscle gets depleted. Due to the glycogen depletion from the muscles, runners are not able to give quality outputs. There are signs of fatigue and feel less competitive. This leads to health problems like losing body protein, electrolytes gets imbalanced, you get dehydrated etc. This is not a sensible way so follow a good diet.

Chapter 15: Factors to consider in Failure in Losing Weight

To enable you to understand how to lose weight effectively it is important to understand why we get fat in the first place. The whole world seems to be getting fat these days with doctors and scientists trying hard to find a solution. In reality the solution is quite simple.

Over the last few decades our diets have turned more and more towards processed foods. Our grandparents were a generation who would buy ingredients to make their food with. They would spend time in the kitchen preparing meals from scratch and they were generally healthy.

Did you know that during WWII in the UK people were healthier than they are today even though they were on rations?

The reason is because people were eating real food and very little else. You may have got hold of some sweets or chocolate but there was very little about. People would grow their own vegetables and could eat as much of that as they liked. With that diet people were lean and physically active.

Fast forward to the 21st century and we are for the most part living on processed food and are generally inactive.

So what is it about processed food that is so bad?

In short processed food typically has several key differences from real food. Let us go through each difference one at a time.

Sugar has been added to almost all processed food which is probably the biggest reason why people are getting fat. When you consume sugar your body increases insulin which in turn forces the energy from the food you have eaten into your fat cells. Basically you get fat.

Another difference is fiber which in processed food is normally removed. It is the fiber which slows down the effects of sugar reducing the amount of insulin and ultimately reducing the amount of energy pushed into your fat cells.

In the real food that our grandparents would eat any food that had sugar which was only fruits and vegetables also had fiber. That meant there was never a problem.

Today sugar has been added to everything including many foods that you wouldn't expect there to be sugar in. Without the fiber our insulin levels remain high and our fat stores continue to grow.

In order to lose weight by running you need to get your eating right first. This means eating real food and cutting out the processed food that you are more than likely currently eating.

You can eat unprocessed meats, fish, eggs, nuts, fruits and vegetables. If man has not played or created it then you can eat it.

What that will do is keep your insulin levels low to none existent. At that point your fat cells will be able to release the stores energy which can then be burnt as you run. The result will be weight loss through a reduced amount of fat; perfect.

You will however need to be aware of a few things that you could fall fowl of. It is what I call The Big Obesity Conspiracy.

For those who have not come across this term before let me tell you a little more about the Big Obesity Conspiracy. I go into more detail in my book but I will summarize it here. You need to know this to ensure you do not fall into the trap.

Modern Times

If you are overweight then you are that way because of what you eat. All weight loss results from the food you eat. While many doctors will say you need to exercise more you can only do that if you eat the right foods.

Eating foods high in sugar as I have already explained will cause your insulin to rise and the energy you have eaten to go into your fat cells. You not only get fatter but you also have no energy left to use.

That means you don't feel like going for a run; you simply don't have the energy. Really you do have the energy but it is all trapped in your fat cells and cannot leave because your insulin levels are preventing it.

As long as you are on a highly processed diet you will not be able to lose weight and maintain it.

As a result of everyone eating a processed food diet and putting on weight all sorts of diets have sprung up. There are hundreds of them all trying to reinvent the wheel.

There is everything from cutting out whole food groups, eating nothing but cabbage, drinking all your food and even eating next to nothing for two days a week.

There are even slimming clubs that get you to buy there branded food disguised as healthy eating but in reality all you are doing is buying a different type of processed food.

Diets do not work; they never have and they never will. Do yourself a favor and stay well clear of them.

Another way that companies will get money out of you on false promises is to get you to buy exercise equipment. This has become a million dollar industry selling all sorts of items to tens of thousands of people each year yet the population continues to get heavier by the year.

You may have purchased an exercise bike to use at home yourself. It has more than likely become a convenient place to hand your ironed shirts.

The problem with this method is it is still buying in to the 'burn more calories than you consume' paradigm. While you do need to burn more calories than you consume this only works if you keep your insulin low. It assumes that calories from sugar are the same as calories from everything else.

This industry sells products because people think they can just burn off the calories. As a wise man once said 'you cannot exercise off a bad diet'. You can however exercise off the fat when you are eating a good one.

Many people also invest in weight loss pills. This is again a bad move. As you now know if you eat an unprocessed diet and exercise you will lose weight. Who needs pills?

Pills actually in many cases have side effects none of which involve losing weight and keeping it off in the long run. They will however result in you losing a whole load of your hard earned cash.

In conclusion the way to eat is to eat fresh unprocessed foods that are low in sugar and high in fiber. I am talking about meat, fish, eggs, nuts, fruits and vegetables. Eat them and exercise and you WILL lose weight.

Ok so you know now that eating right and exercise will result in weight loss we need to do the mathematics behind it.

Each pound of fat no matter where it is on your body has a total of 3500 calories. This means that if for example you need to lose 10 pounds in weight you simply multiply 3500 by 10 giving 35,000. So to lose that much weight you need to burn 35,000 more than you consume. Simple enough isn't it?

Once you have the number of calories you need to lose you can work out how many you want to lose a day. To keep things simple let us say it is 500 a day; that would mean you would lose 1 pound a week. You can then set your food and exercise accordingly.

It is calories burnt less calories consumed to give you your weight loss. Calories burnt are a total of active metabolic rate and exercise combined.

You start this by working out your active metabolic rate. Now you may have heard of basic metabolic rate but you may not have heard of active. Let me explain.

Basic Metabolic Rate in case you don't know will give you the number of calories your body will burn each day just keeping you alive. It assumes you do nothing but exist.

Active metabolic rate takes into account the fact that you get out of bed, you may go up and down stairs, do the hovering, go to work and so on.

Knowing how many calories you burn in a day can never be 100% but you can get it close.

People who pull you toward negative instant gratification decisions or activities that directly conflict with your fitness and weight loss goals are drain people.

Don't tax your willpower unnecessarily. Eliminate or avoid drain people as much as possible.

When you can't avoid drain people, seek to minimize their impact by making your goals clear and willpower evident. Typically, drain people want to hang out with like-minded people and don't want to be reminded of their own shortcomings or lack of fitness motivation.

Remember, you only have so much willpower available in a 24-hour period before your willpower starts to wane and become more difficult to maintain due to declining energy or sleepiness.

Be careful of overworking and overtraining because it can lead to burnout. Symptoms of burnout include a noticeable decline in motivation, willpower, performance, and results. Adhering to this warning and avoiding burnout is typically difficult for uninformed "Type A" personalities and perfectionists who want to apply willpower to every task throughout the entire day.

Remember—for the best long-term results, you should conserve your willpower for daily decisions and activities that will directly impact your crucial fitness goals. Don't waste precious willpower energy on insignificant goals.

Fact: Drugs, medications, and alcohol can impair mental capacity and weaken your willpower. If you want to conserve willpower and fitness motivation, do not ingest or abuse mind-altering substances.

When I was losing weight I used the calculations found in one of Jillian Michaels books. It can also be found on her website. It allows you to work out what you burn each day. See below.

We have often heard that running is the best form of exercising. The truth is not far from it. Running is definitely one of the best ways to lose weight and one of the healthiest options for the wellbeing of your body. However, it is not as simple as it seems. You need to focus your energy in the right manner towards running if you want to get the best results.

Chapter 16: Achieving the Lasting Fitness

Once you have made the decision to take responsibility for your fitness and weight loss—does this mean that you are committed?

The assumption of commitment by way of responsibility is a mistaken notion that many people accept. My goal is to help you become a fitness motivation master, so you must learn and internalize the fact that taking charge and accepting responsibility are crucial steps along your path to fitness success. You must also learn that taking charge and accepting responsibility are not the same as commitment.

Think of those instances in your life when you have seen someone volunteer to take charge or accept responsibility for something that, in the end, did not achieve the desired results. Maybe they began extremely gung-ho, yet somewhere along the line their motivation, enthusiasm, and energy faded and their effectiveness suffered. There are even those who have volunteered to take charge and who never show up! Something occurred between the time they made the decision to accept responsibility and the time it came to execute.

After you have accepted responsibility for your fitness, weight loss, and health--it is time to make a conscious commitment to the fitness lifestyle!

Take a Courage to Commit

In order to achieve the fitness you want this is the most essential thing you need, commitment. Commitment is a state or quality of dedication. To be committed is to be obligated to something and willing to give 100%---not 80 or 90%--but, 100% focus and effort.

You must commit fully to the fitness lifestyle if you want to maximize your fitness motivation and physical results.

For fitness motivation masters, commitment is expressed as a conviction. For those lacking sufficient belief, commitment is typically expressed as a "wish" or "hope."

Most people don't make strong decisions or declarations. They state weak preferences. Preferences can be altered, ignored, or changed. Preferences are exceptionally vulnerable to excuses, adverse challenges, or circumstances.

You must "go all out" to truly separate yourself from the crowd. A decisive commitment is one where you leave no doubt about your conviction and future actions.

Now that you know that you are in charge of your fitness success---it is imperative that you fully commit to achieving it. Commitment is vitally important for anyone who wants to achieve a significant goal. A firm commitment makes fitness motivation easier and more sustainable.

Practice demonstrating commitment regularly. The best way to do this is to invest time, resources, and energy into the behaviors and activities that will deliver the desired results in fitness and weight loss. Stop investing in activities, things, or people that do not result in consistent progress toward your fitness and weight loss goals.

Keep in mind that commitment does not guarantee constant success. Fitness motivation masters may fail along the way to success, but they do not make excuses (remember, you must accept responsibility). You may occasionally falter in your journey to success, but you will learn to identify the true reasons for progress impairment—and you will learn to take immediate steps to correct bad decisions and behavioral mistakes.

For most people--real commitment is simple in principle, but hard to put into practice. For starters, I suggest you just commit that you will not give up—and that you will persist in gaining the knowledge, motivation, support, and tools to reach your fitness and weight loss goals. I've witnessed many clients experience a breakthrough in their fitness and weight loss, once they made a no-excuse commitment to success!

Success in fitness or weight loss does not often come immediately or even on the first try, but a commitment to the process will prevent you from "dropping out" of the process—which will ultimately lead to you achieving your goals faster.

Lifestyle Modification

It is not enough that you just simply commit but take it into actions is all that matters. The fitness lifestyle is the enjoyable pursuit of optimum health and physical performance. A fitness lifestyle fuels and maximizes your fitness motivation.

To live a fitness lifestyle you must commit to move beyond temporary fitness or weight loss solutions. You must commit to developing personal habits that support a fitness lifestyle and physical transformation. If you are unwilling to commit to a fitness lifestyle, you will be unwilling to make the choices and decisions needed to sustain fitness motivation and lasting physical results.

Any weight loss strategy that focuses only on weight loss will eventually fail. By committing to a fitness lifestyle, you will automatically lose weight. More importantly, you will finally keep it off. Fitness motivation masters happily embrace this fact. Conversely, yo-yo dieters and sporadic fitness enthusiasts consistently fail to accept the fact that commitment to the fitness lifestyle is the most successful path to fitness and permanent weight loss.

For the purpose of achieving fitness and weight loss success, there are two major components of the fitness lifestyle.

1. Effective management of your diet.

2. Effective management of your physical activity.

Below are the seven consistent behaviors of fitness motivation masters based on my observation and study of clients who have successfully achieved their target fitness and weight loss goals—and maintained their goals for more than one year.

1. Resolve and purpose (commitment).

2. Positive "can-do" attitude.

3. Healthy eating habits.

4. Active lifestyle.

5. Regular results tracking.

6. Willingness to accept full responsibility for success and failure.

7. Consistently seeking more knowledge on fitness and weight management.

If you want it grab it

They said that will power is the key that drive people to achieve what they want. A growing body of evidence indicates that willpower and self-control are essential for a happy and healthy life. As a fitness motivation student, you must learn how to develop and maximize willpower and self-control, so that you can resist negative influences and eliminate bad habits that undermine your fitness and weight management.

We have many common names for willpower: self-control, impulse control, delayed gratification, resolve, or determination. According to most psychological scientists, willpower can be described as follows:

* The ability to delay gratification, resisting short-term temptations in order to achieve long-term goals.

* The capacity to override an unwanted or negative thought, feeling or impulse.

* The ability to employ a "rational" cognitive system of behavior rather than an "irrational" emotional system.

* Conscious regulation of the self by the self.

* A limited resource capable of being depleted.

Motivation (covered in the previous chapter) is about increasing desire to do something that moves you closer toward your goals. Whereas, willpower is more about having the skills and ability to resist or not do something that conflicts with and undermines progress toward your goals.

Two main areas of the brain contribute to the process of willpower-- the limbic system (located right under the brain) and the prefrontal cortex (the front section of the brain right behind your forehead). These sections of the brain are linked closely together, and their communication efficiency determines how well you can exhibit willpower and self-control.

The limbic system is the "emotional" part of the brain. It is associated with your desires and urges for instant gratification. The prefrontal cortex is the "logical" part of the brain, which is associated with the cognitive function of rational thought, decision-making, and behavior regulation.

Whenever an emotional response is generated by the limbic system, the prefrontal cortex then interprets the response. This allows the prefrontal cortex to produce a logical behavioral response based on the situation. The more active your prefrontal cortex is--the greater your capacity for willpower and emotional control.

The willpower process is activated in response to an internal conflict. Let's use lunchtime as an example. The desire for instant gratification may cause an individual to order a supersized fast food lunch, followed by a cigarette break. Conversely, motivation and a stronger desire to exercise willpower may cause an individual to order a healthy and hearty salad, followed by a short walk.

One of the most consistent scientific findings about willpower is that it seems to be finite—that is, we only have so much during a 24-hour period and it runs out as we use it—and we need to replenish it regularly. Willpower depends on the body's natural energy cycle and tends to be strongest at the beginning of the day.

Trying to control your instant gratification desires, negative emotions, non-vital distractions, or simply refusing an unhealthy desert all tap the same source of mental strength known as willpower. The more we use willpower, the weaker it tends to get throughout the day.

Willpower is essentially like a muscle—it can be exhausted by overuse, but just like our physical muscles--researchers believe we can strengthen our willpower and expand its capacity by training it. Because willpower is like a muscle--you have to exhaust it in the short-term in order to build its strength in the long-term.

Your willpower is strengthened by doing anything that gets your brain out of its comfort zone in a healthy manner. When you actively work to develop your fitness motivation and health habits, you deplete your willpower in the process--but over time, the strength of your willpower increases--making you better able to demonstrate fitness motivation consistency for achieving your goals in the future.

Improving your Desire to Improve

The best part about creating a new willpower habit is that not only does it strengthen your Motivate Fit skills--it also frees up more of your willpower for other things. When a decision evolves into a habit--it draws little, if any, energy from your willpower supply. The more healthy decisions and actions you can make habitual, the less impact and drain on your willpower you'll experience throughout the day.

This is why Motivate Fit students with stronger self-control actually spend less time resisting desires than those with weaker self-control. By developing willpower, fitness motivation, and good habits— motivate Fit students can minimize the number of temptations they face by making daily fitness decisions and actions automatic.

In order to increase your willpower, you must learn to enjoy the moments and process of exercising and strengthening your willpower. This attitude and approach to willpower development will help you reach your fitness goals faster and maintain your success longer.

If you are going to be a highly fit individual for life--you must fall in love with the destination (goal), and you must fall in love with traveling the actual journey (which is the process of developing willpower and other fitness motivation skills).

Use the pleasure of seeing yourself growing and developing unstoppable willpower as added motivation to continue exercising your willpower until it becomes automatic. When I was first learning how to strengthen my willpower, I would pat myself on the back (literally) and say "great job" every time I exercised willpower throughout the day.

I suggest you use this simple reinforcing tool. You can insert your name to make it feel even more personal. And, don't worry if you are reluctant about shouting to yourself in a crowded room. You can pat yourself on the back and silently tell yourself that you did a "great job" whenever you exercise willpower.

You can also use the pain of potentially seeing yourself fall short of maximizing your potential as motivation to exercise regular willpower and ensure significant progress toward your goals.

Do not fall victim to the bad advice that you should reward yourself (associate pleasure) with the very things that you will use willpower to avoid or stop doing. The problem with this bad advice—for example, having a piece of chocolate cake to reward yourself for losing three pounds this week—is that it undermines the development and optimization of your willpower and fitness motivation habits.

Inevitably, you will experience lapses as you are developing your willpower and self-control skills. But, please make the following promise to yourself: Never say—"oh well forget it" or allow yourself to spiral out of control just because you lose one episode of "willpower vs. instant gratification."

Motivate students—and even world-class athletes--have occasional lapses in willpower. The difference between motivated students (or professional athletes) and the average person is that there willpower lapses are much less frequent (perhaps once every month or maybe once every week—as opposed to once every day or even once every hour for those with nonexistent willpower).

Motivated students typically have willpower lapses on things that are not critical to their key goals. Whereas, those with low self-control skills will experience consistent willpower lapses on important decisions and actions related to their key goals.

Because willpower is a real, finite energy, the question that naturally arises is; how can you conserve and strengthen this force to maximize your fitness motivation skills?

How do you generate enough willpower energy to strive towards and achieve success? The first step is to consciously conserve this energy, by keeping it from being squandered--and saving it for the fitness and weight loss goals that are most important and impactful to you.

Know Your Goals

Because willpower is a finite resource—chasing too many goals at once will drain your mental strength, and will not provide sufficient willpower for any of your goals. The result is typically failure in most, if not all of your goals. Instead, you should funnel your willpower towards one or two key fitness goals at any given time.

Clear goals provide clear focus for your brain and added motivation to exercise your willpower. If you set S.M.A.R.T. (specific, measurable, actionable, realistic, and_timed) goals—you will be ten times more likely to reach your goals than those who have poorly articulated or "non-smart" goals.

Proper Preparation

Science and daily life have both provided ample evidence that planners are winners. This is why I've incorporated this crucial element into the motivate Fit Method.

You cannot achieve sustainable success of any significant measure without learning how to properly plan and prepare. Plans don't need to be complicated. Often, it's the simplest plans that are most effective.

The definition of luck is when preparation meets opportunity. If you learn to appreciate, enjoy, and invest in planning and preparation--

you will excel in fitness, weight management, and all areas of your life.

Live Simply

Simplicity is a constant and trustworthy companion for all peak performers in life. Simplification leads to less clutter in your mind, which helps to conserve your valuable willpower.

Following are some recommendations to help you simplify your life and mind to better support your fitness and weight loss goals.

Plan ahead of time

Whenever you recognize a specific and necessary decision or activity that demands repetition—begin to seek out ways to automate the task. This will free up time and mental energy. The best way make a task more efficient varies, but options include--technology solutions; improved processes; and delegation or outsourcing.

You should evaluate any repetitive task occasionally and ask yourself if it is necessary. If a task is simply not necessary, eliminate it.

Lists everything

Lists are a very effective way to save time and free up your mind power for more critical tasks. Using lists will improve your productivity and effectiveness. Every successful individual has learned how to use lists to help manage performance and deliver superior results.

You can choose to keep important lists (such as a healthy diet grocery list) in your smartphone, or you can simply use pen and paper.

Organized Everything

Highly successful and fit people place a high value on their time. A commitment to becoming and staying organized will save time and reduce stress, which makes it easier to use your willpower for fitness and weight loss.

Chronic disorganization will deplete your willpower. Simplify your life and protect your mental energy by implementing simple routines to stay organized at home, work, school, and during travel.

Sleep

Sleep is a natural periodic state of unconscious rest for the mind and body. Adequate sleep is vital to willpower functioning, fitness motivation, and sports performance.

The most successful athletes and motivate Fit students make time for adequate sleep and rest. Being well-rested will have a positive impact on your fitness motivation and physical performance.

Sleep improves split-second decision-making ability by 4.3%.

Tennis players get a 42% boost in hitting accuracy when they get adequate sleep.

An athlete's maximum bench press drops by 20 pounds after four days of inadequate sleep.

Similar outcomes related to sleeping habits were found when observing and testing business executives. The more rested they were, the better they performed on cognitive skill tests and decision-making assessments.

Research suggests that even small amounts of sleep deprivation will take a significant toll on your health, mood, cognitive capacity, and productivity. Conserving, exercising, and managing willpower becomes exponentially harder as sleep deprivation increases.

Don't fool yourself by bragging to your colleagues and friends about how you can function on a few hours of sleep per night! Champion athletes and highly fit individuals understand the importance and power of this most basic human function. Sleep is much more important than your ego!

LeBron James is one of the most celebrated and gifted professional athletes in professional sports today. In addition to innate talent and dedicated training—LeBron credits healthy sleeping habits as one of the keys to his peak performance consistency.

During particularly intense periods, such as during the playoffs-- LeBron often sleeps up to 12 hours a day. This may seem like a lot for most people, but elite athletes place an enormous amount of stress on their bodies and minds—which requires significant sleep time for complete repair and recuperation.

As a motivated student—you should get adequate sleep each night if you want to conserve your willpower and keep your fitness motivation functioning at a high level.

Naps are a natural and powerful willpower conservation tool that you can use when you don't have a lot of time for regular sleep--or simply need a boost in physical or mental energy. Short, effective naps can be as little as five minutes--and longer, more restorative naps can be as long as ninety minutes.

For most elite athletes—exercise is part of their job. For anyone outside of sports—consistent exercise and healthy eating have been linked to increased willpower. In essence, willpower improves your fitness—and as your fitness improves, you will gain increased willpower. It's a really nice "circle of success!"

Certainly, you will be better equipped to conserve and exercise willpower if you are effectively managing your stress and mood. Recent studies have shown that exercise is effective in reducing stress and even short-term bouts of depression.

Suffering from a known or unknown physical or mental ailment can have an adverse effect on your willpower and fitness motivation. I recommend scheduling regular physical exams with a medical doctor. You should view your doctor as a key member of your fitness motivation success team.

Keep on The track of your To Do List

Remember, our goal is to make sure you get the highest return on your investment of willpower each day by applying your limited mind energy to your top one or two fitness goals. This ensures that you will get better results and make faster progress.

You can reach your fitness and weight loss goals more quickly if you take the time to evaluate your performance and results on a regular basis. Using this proven strategy--you will always know what's working and what's not working to help you exercise and eat right more consistently.

By knowing the key drivers of your success—you can focus your willpower on those decisions and activities that are proving to be most beneficial.

Conclusion

Achieving the fitness you always dream of is not an easy tasks. It need enough knowledge and determination to arrive at your goals. I hope this book helps you to achieve this goal. All of the information in this book are geared towards the improvement not only physical fitness but fitness as whole of a person.

Many of us think that being fit is all about achieving a right body but without proper mindset to maintain it it will eventually wane out and you will eventually lose the fight for better healthy living. This book promotes an overall healthy lifestyle for a better lifestyle.

Being fit does not require rigid regimen but rather discovering what you truly love and able to enjoy and live as healthy as you should be. Don't be fooled that they are always easy way out because there are none. I hope this book enlighten your mind about the right ways to achieve the fitness you truly deserved.

www.ingramcontent.com/pod-product-compliance
Lightning Source LLC
Chambersburg PA
CBHW062010280526
45787CB00005B/2050